Care of Eyes

Care of Eyes

By
DR J. AGARWAL
DR T. AGARWAL

Edited by:
DR SUNITA AGARWAL
DR ATHIYA AGARWAL
DR AMAR AGARWAL

Rupa & Co

Copyright © Dr J. Agarwal and Dr Mrs T. Agarwal 2002

First Published 2002
Third Impression 2010

Published by
Rupa Publications India Pvt. Ltd.
7/16, Ansari Road, Daryaganj
New Delhi 110 002

Sales Centres:
Allahabad Bengaluru Chandigarh Chennai
Hyderabad Jaipur Kathmandu
Kolkata Mumbai

All rights reserved.
No part of this publication may be reproduced, stored in a retrieval system, or transmitted, in any form or by any means, electronic, mechanical, photocopying, recording or otherwise, without the prior permission of the publishers.

Typeset in 12 pts. Caxton by
Mindways Design
1410 Chiranjiv Tower
43 Nehru Place
New Delhi 110 019

Printed in India by
Gopsons Papers Ltd.
A-14 Sector 60
Noida 201 301

Contents

Introduction	ix
Normal Eye	1
Refractive Errors	6
Contact Lenses	32
Zyoptix Laser/Lasik Laser	36
Headache	47
Red Eye	49
Cataract	53

Glaucoma	78
Eye Transplantation	84
Squint	87
Diabetes	91
Retinal Detachment and other Retinal Diseases	97
Injuries and Deficiency Diseases	103
Hints	106
General Instructions	110
Important Signs and Symptoms	112

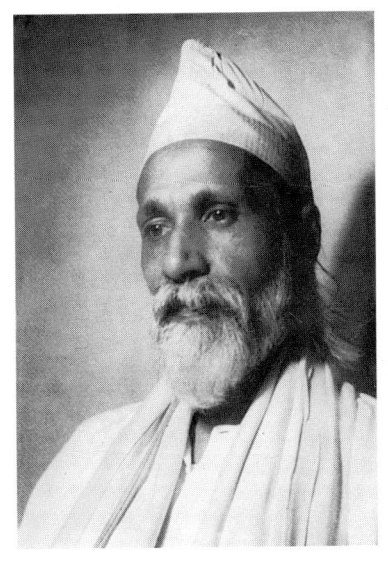

*Dedicated to
Our Father Dr R.S. Agarwal
(1900-1974)
The Discoverer of a Synthesis in Ophthalmic Science*

Introduction

Eyes are the best gift of nature to the body. One is not even aware of their importance as long as the vision is perfect. It is only when one's sight begins to fail that one realises with a shock the importance of the eyes.

Throughout the ages, blindness and diseases leading to blindness have been regarded as a part of human destiny, but such an attitude of fatalism cannot be accepted today. It must be admitted that certain forms of blindness are not preventable and some cannot be cured or even arrested. Fortunately, the number of such diseases is declining. In most cases blindness is caused by preventable diseases and unnecessary accidents which can be avoided if a little precaution is observed. There are many more cases where medical or surgical measures can restore vision. Preservation of good eyesight is almost impossible without eye-health education.

To a child born blind, the beauties of life and nature do not exist. Whereas to a person who has known the restless waves of the ocean, the multi-coloured butterflies and flowers, birds flying over the mountains and green valleys — loss of sight is a tragedy without any parallel. Therefore, those who are gifted with sight need constant and vigilant care of their eyes to conserve vision and restore it if need be. Moreover, the cost of preventing a disease is only a fraction of the amount spent on the treatment of the disease once it has set in, as a colossal amount is needed for the rehabilitation of the blind.

It is with this idea that this book has been written so that the reader may know the proper eye-care methods and apply them in order to prevent a needless loss of sight. Thus the coming of total night may be prevented before the eyes close forever.

Dr J. Agarwal
Dr T. Agarwal

Normal Eye

The eye resembles a Camera. Just as we take a photograph with a camera, the eye takes a photograph of an object seen by it. In the camera, an object is focused on the film of the camera by a lens (Fig. 1). This image is an inverted image and it is developed in the studio and made into an erect one. In the same way, an object is focused by the lens of the eye on the film of the eye called the **Retina**. This image is also inverted and is made erect by the brain.

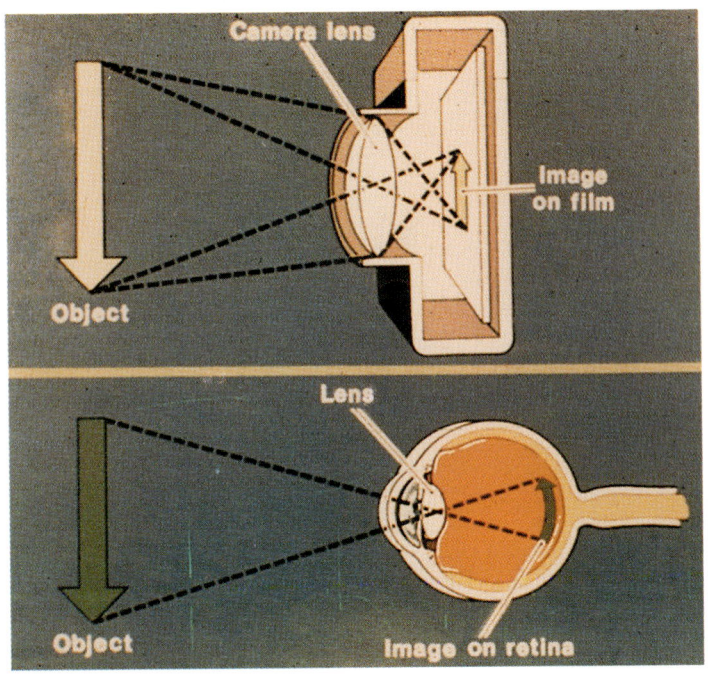

Figure 1: Optics of a camera and an eye are similar. The top figure shows the optics of a camera. An object is focused by the camera lens on to the film of the camera. The image is thus formed on the film which is then sent to the studio for developing. The image is inverted and the studio then erects the image. The normal eye works in the same fashion. This can be seen in the bottom figure. The object is focused by the lens of the eye on to the retina. The retina is like the film of the camera. The image of the object which is inverted is focused on to the retina. The image is then sent via the nerve of the eye (optic nerve) to the best studio in the world which is the human brain. There the brain automatically erects the image.

Let us look at a cross-section of the eye to understand its various parts. The **Eyelids** cover our eye and there

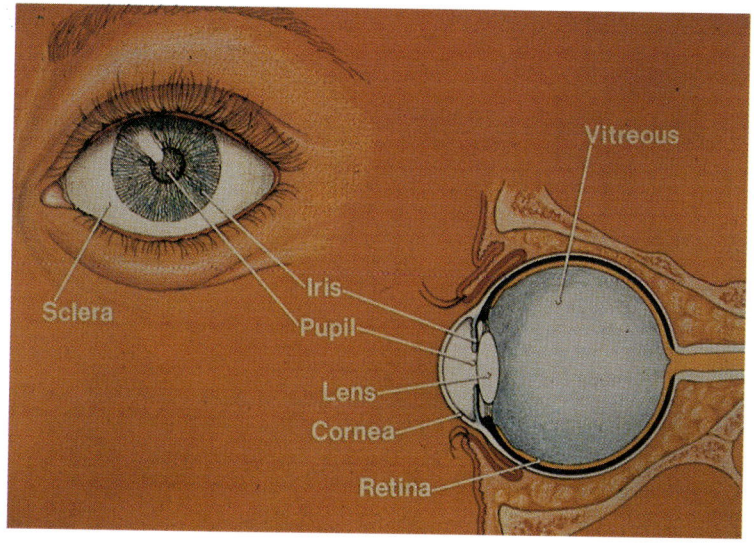

Figure 2: Anatomy of the human eye. The figure on the left shows the eye as we see it. The figure on the right shows a cross-section of the eye showing the inner structures of the eye.

is a thin membrane covering the inner aspect of the lids and the front part of the sclera called the **Conjunctiva**. The eye has an outer window called the **Cornea**. This allows light to enter through it and so it is transparent (Figs. 2 and 3.). There is a fluid in the eye between the cornea and the lens called the **Aqueous Humor**. Just as the camera has a diaphragm, the eye has a diaphragm which controls the amount of light entering the eye. This is called **Iris**. It has a small aperture in the centre for light to pass through, called the **Pupil**. When it is

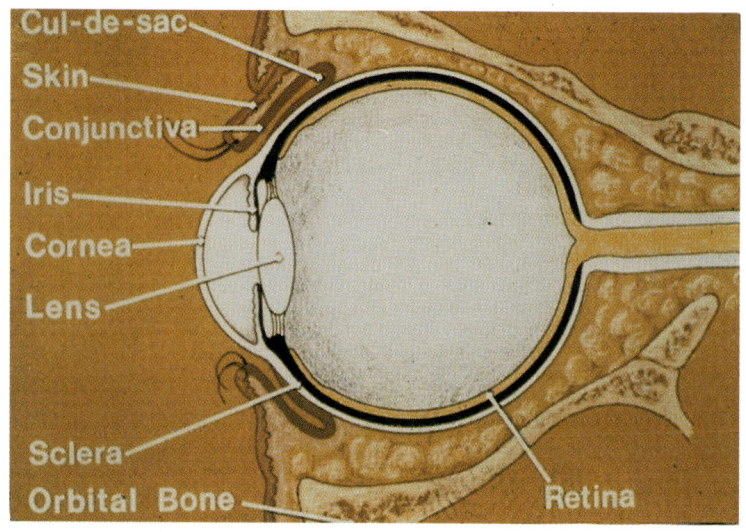

Figure 3: Cross-section of the eye.

day and the eye needs little light to pass into it, the iris constricts and the pupil becomes small. When it is night and the eye needs more light to pass through it the iris expands and the pupil becomes larger (dilates). There is a viscous liquid between the lens and the retina which forms the contour of the eye called the **Vitreous Body**. The retina gets its nourishment from the **Choroid** and the outermost post of all is a thick coat of the eye called the **Sclera** which protects the eye from injury. The impulses from the retina reach the brain by a nerve of the eye called the **Optic Nerve**. This is seen as the Optic disc which is next to the macula. The most important portion of the retina is the **Macula** which contributes to 90% of our vision (Fig. 4) and helps us achieve fine vision.

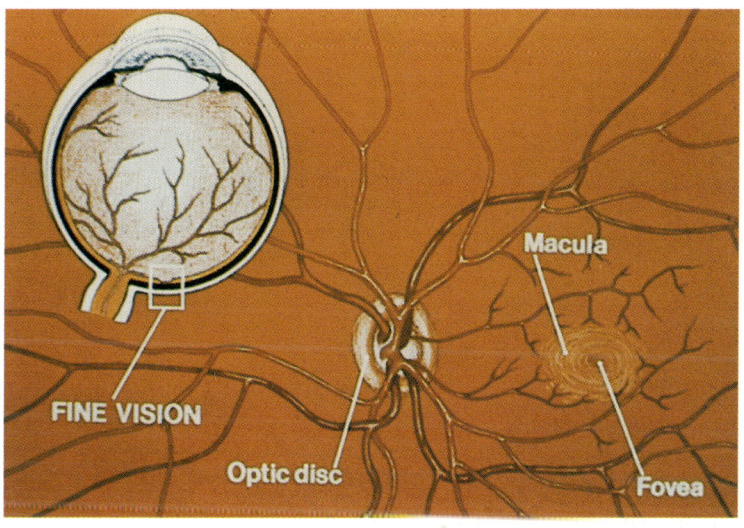

Figure 4: Macula of the eye. The macula is the area of the retina (film of the eye) which helps us achieve fine vision.

Refractive Errors

What are Refractive Errors?

The eye is a sense organ and functions like any other sense organ. Just as we smell and hear, so also do we see. No efforts are made to hear and smell, similarly, the eye does not make an effort to see when it functions normally. Some people are not able to see clearly and only with the help of spectacles are able to see clearly. The inabilty to see clearly without spectacles is called a **Refractive Error**. Patients suffering from refractive errors see clearly only with the help of spectacles.

Types of Refractive Errors

1. Myopia or Short-sightedness.
2. Hypermetropia or Long-sightedness.
3. Astigmatism.
4. Presbyopia.
5. Aberropia

Myopia or Short-sightedness

Short-sightedness means an inability to see at a distance. In other words for near (short) vision, the vision is perfect but when the person tries to see distant (long) objects there is difficulty. In a normal eye, the cornea and lens will bend the light perfectly in order to focus exactly on the retina. This is the light-sensitive layer at the back of the eye. It is where the image of what we see is formed (Fig. 5). Numerous light-sensitive receptors called **rods** and **cones** are found here. These structures are responsible for giving colour and contrast to our vision. People who suffer from myopia have eyes longer than normal or the cornea is too curved. As a result, light rays are focused to form an image at a

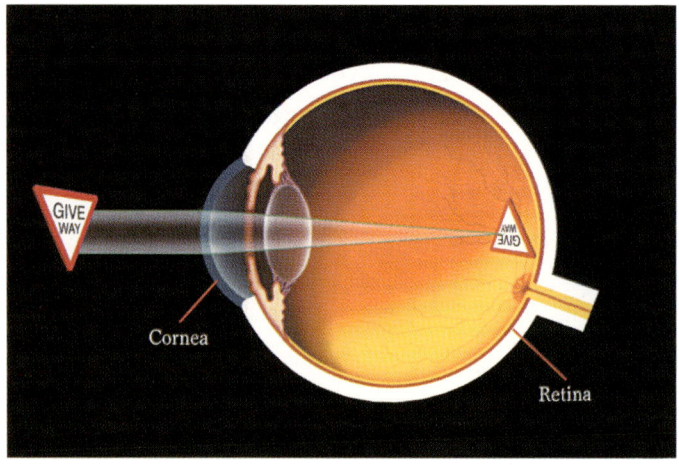

Figure 5: Normal vision. The image is focused on the retina.
(*Courtesy:* Dr Jerry tan, Singapore)

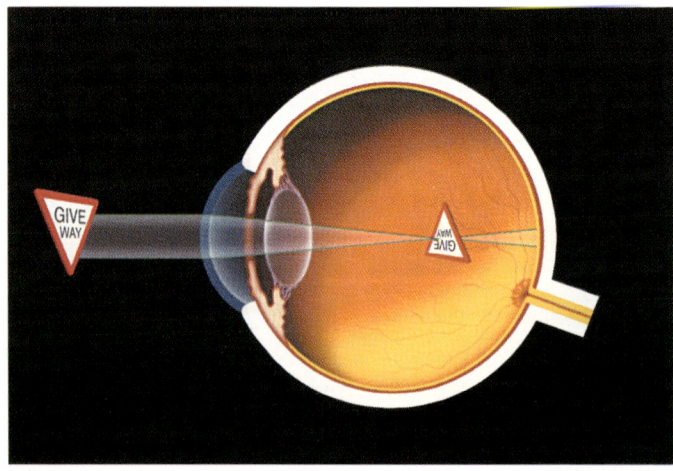

Figure 6: Myopic eye. The object is focused in front of the retina.
(*Courtesy*. Dr Jerry Tan, Singapore)

point before the retina (Fig.6). Hence, our brain perceives it as a blurred image. As the object is moved closer to our eye, it becomes clearer and more defined as the image moves towards the retina. This movement towards the retina brings the image into better focus (Fig. 7). As the image of the object is focused in front of the retina (Fig. 8), to correct it one has to use a spectacle which has the power to divert the rays of light more so that the image is focused on the retina. This is done with the help of a **Concave Lens** or a **Minus Lens** (Fig. 9).

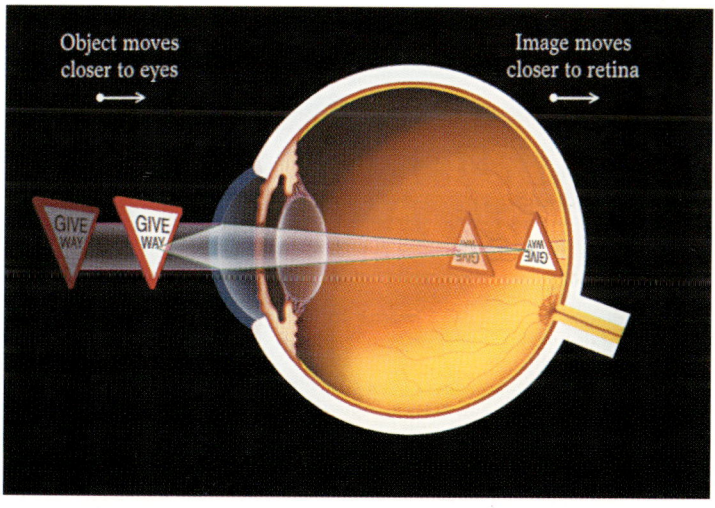

Figure 7: Myopic eye. If the object is brought closer to the eye the image falls on the retina and the patient can see well. This is why a myopic patient can see near objects clearly but not distant objects.
(*Courtesy:* Dr Jerry Tan, Singapore)

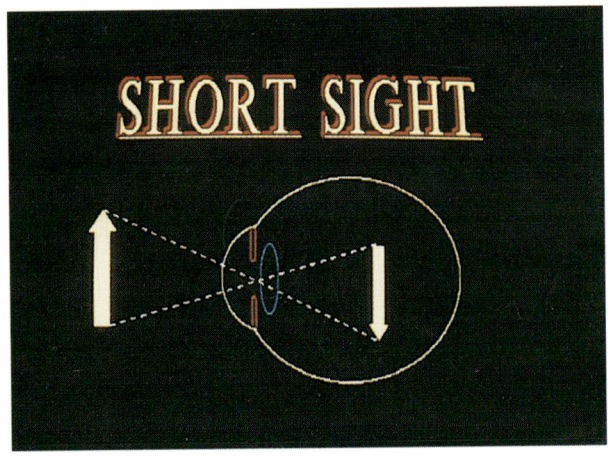

Figure 8: Short sight (myopia). The eyeball is longer than normal, so the image of the object falls in front of the retina.

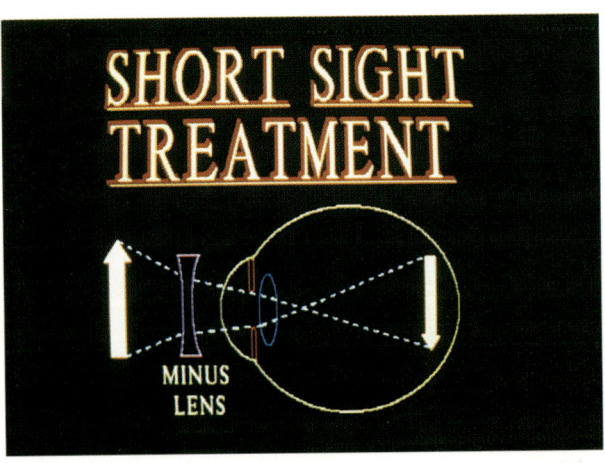

Figure 9: Short sight treatment. Minus lenses or concave lenses will diverge the rays of light so that the image falls on the retina and the patient sees well. That is why myopic patients wear minus lenses.

Hypermetropia or Long-sightedness

Long-sightedness means an inability to see near objects. Long-sighted people can see distant (long) objects clearly. They have shorter than normal eyes or corneas which are too flat. So, the image of the object is focused behind the retina (Fig. 10). Objects at a greater distance are slightly blurred while objects seen at a nearer distance are more blurred (Fig. 11). To correct this problem (Fig. 12) one has to use a spectacle which has the power to converge the rays of light so that the image is focused on the retina. This is done with the help of a **Convex Lens** or a **Plus Lens**. (Fig. 13).

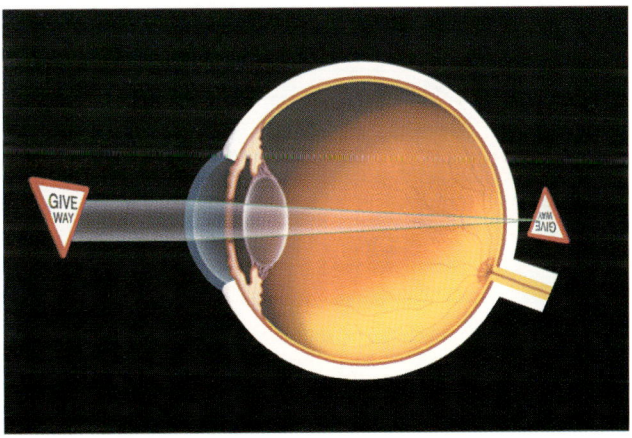

Figure 10: Hyperopic Eye. The object is focused behind the retina.
(*Courtesy*: Dr Jerry Tan, Singapore)

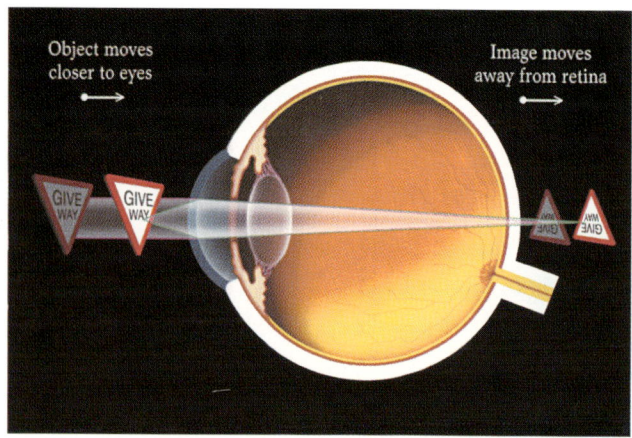

Figure 11: Hyperopic Eye. If the object is brought closer to the eye the image goes further behind the retina and the patient sees even less. This is why a hyperopic patient cannot see near objects clearly. (*Courtesy:* Dr Jerry Tan, Singapore)

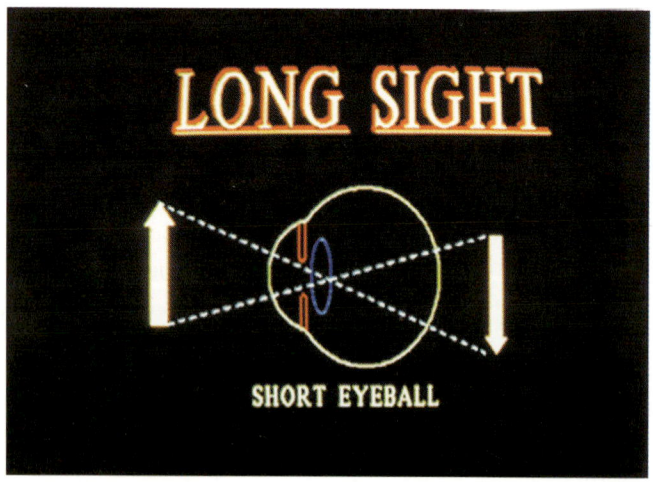

Figure 12: Long sight (Hyperopia). The eye ball is shorter than normal so the image of the object falls behind the retina.

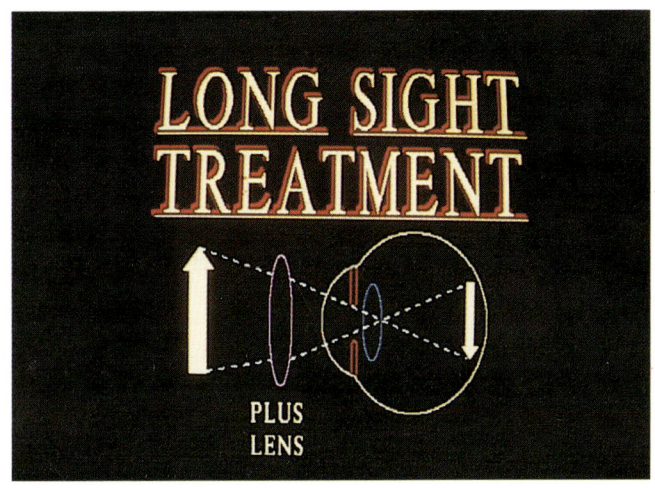

Figure 13: Long sight treatment. Plus lenses or convex lenses will converge the rays of light so that the image falls on to the retina and the patient sees well. That is why hyperopic patients wear plus lenses.

Astigmatism

If one axis of the object is focused well on the retina (for example, the vertical axis) and the other axis (for example, the horizontal axis) is not focused onto the retina the condition is called **Astigmatism**. To treat this one has to use spectacles (with cylindrical lenses) only for the axis which is defective.

Normally, our cornea has a surface similar to that of a smooth spherical ball like the side of a bowling ball (Fig 14). However, when the cornea takes the shape

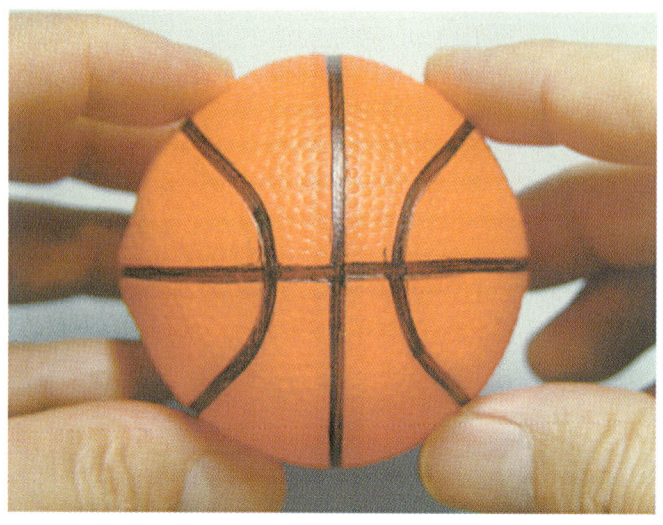

Figure 14: Spherical surface of a ball. The normal cornea is like this.
(*Courtesy*: Dr Jerry Tan, Singapore)

of a dessert spoon, it produces a condition called astigmatism, where light rays are haphazardly focused at different points in the eye, distorting the vision. If we take an example of a smooth spherical ball it will be abnormally shaped (Fig. 15). Most people have regular astigmatism, which means that the surface of the eye has two curvatures. Light focuses on one point from one curvature while the other curvature focuses light on another point (Fig. 16). Images are thus doubled giving the appearance of shadowing or multiple images as many people with astigmatism complain (Figs. 17 and 18).

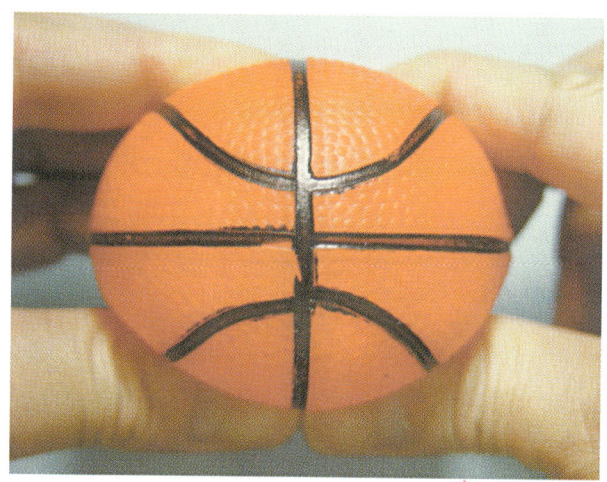

Figure 15: Abnormally shaped ball. The astigmatic cornea looks like this.
(*Courtesy*: Dr Jerry Tan, Singapore)

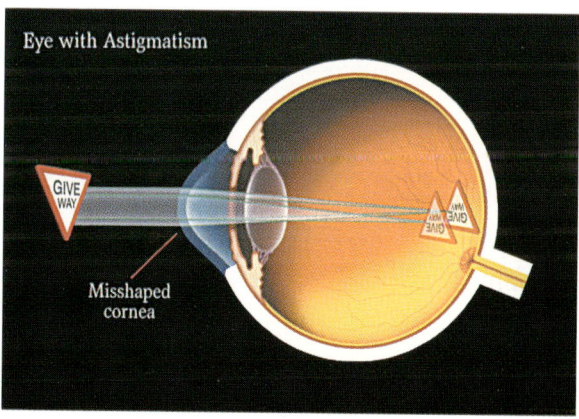

Figure 16: Eye with astigmatism. In an eye with astigmatism, light rays are improperly bent and are focused at several points on the retina. Some areas of vision may be clear, while others may be blurred or distorted.
(*Courtesy*: Dr Jerry Tan, Singapore)

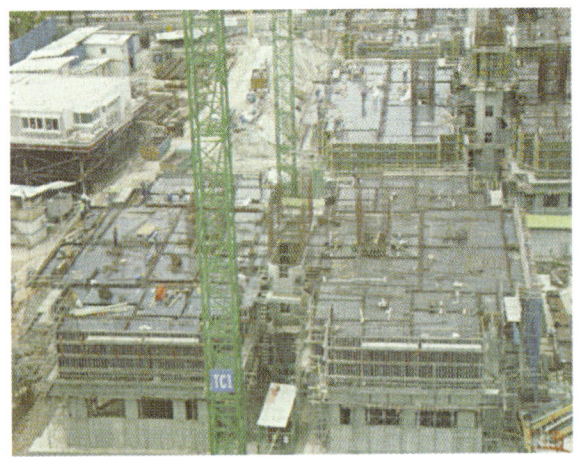

Figure 17: An eye with no astigmatism sees a clear image.
(*Courtesy:* Dr Jerry Tan, Singapore)

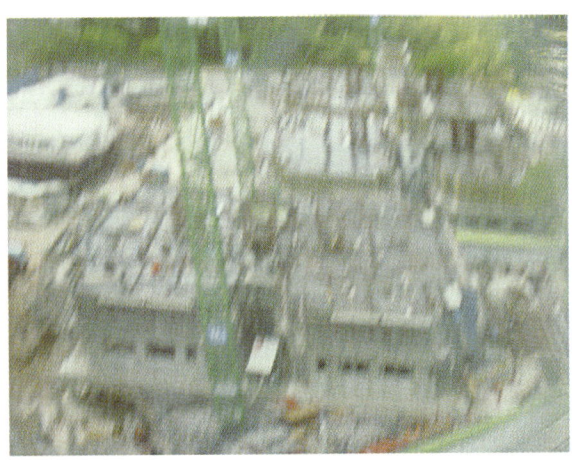

Figure 18: An eye with astigmatism sees a blurred image.
(*Courtesy:* Dr Jerry Tan, Singapore)

Presbyopia

When we use a camera and focus on a distant object we turn the lens so that the image is focused on the film. Then when we want to photograph a near object the lens has again to be rotated to change the focusing. The same happens with our eye. When we see a distant object the lens automatically focuses and suddenly when we focus onto the lettering of this book the lens automatically refocuses to get this near object (lettering of the book) focused on the retina. In other words our eye works like an **Auto-focusing Camera**. This system works till we reach forty years of age. After that the eye starts getting older and does not focus by itself. This is because the lens starts getting harder and does not auto-focus. So, by the time we reach forty years our distant vision may be allright but for us to visualise a near object like reading this book we have to use a convex lens or plus lens. This refractive error is called **Presbyopia** (Figs. 19 and 20).

The difference between Presbyopia and Hypermetropia is that in Presbyopia, it is the lens that is at fault and not the shape of the eye or cornea. Furthermore, for Presbyopia, the eyes have a fixed focus, which means the eyes can only focus within a narrow range of vision.

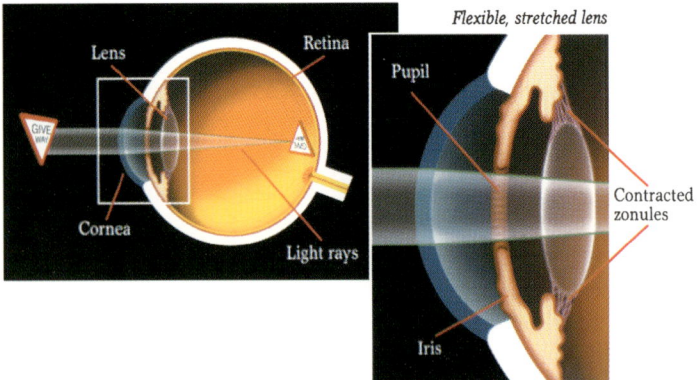

Figure 19: Normal eye focuses distant and near objects. When we look at a near object, the brain sends impulses to the focusing muscles of the eye to contract and relax the zonules. This contraction and relaxation adjust the shape of the lens, focusing the images on the retina.
(*Courtesy:* Dr Jerry Tan, Singapore)

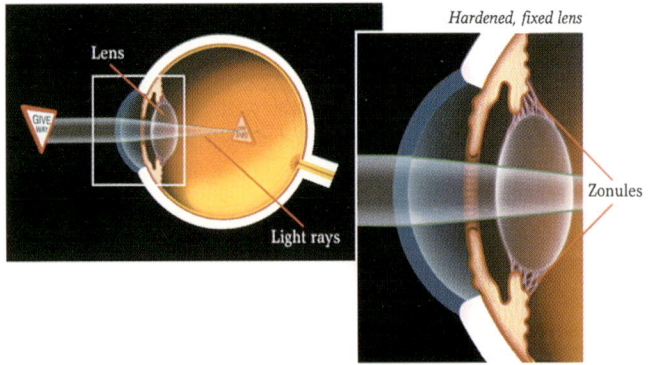

Figure 20: Presbyopic eye. As we get older, especially after the age of 40 years, the human lens begins to harden and the ability to change its shape becomes more difficult. The focusing of images becomes less efficient, especially for near objects. This is called presbyopia.
(*Courtesy:* Dr Jerry Tan, Singapore)

Aberropia

This is a new refractive error discovered recently. In this, aberrations are present in the eye which produce less vision and patients are generally diagnosed as suffering from Amblyopia or lazy eyes. They actually suffer from Aberropia.

Computerised Eye Testing

A lot is heard regarding computerised eye testing. This is done by means of a computer which automatically tells one the power of the eye (Fig. 21). It is called an

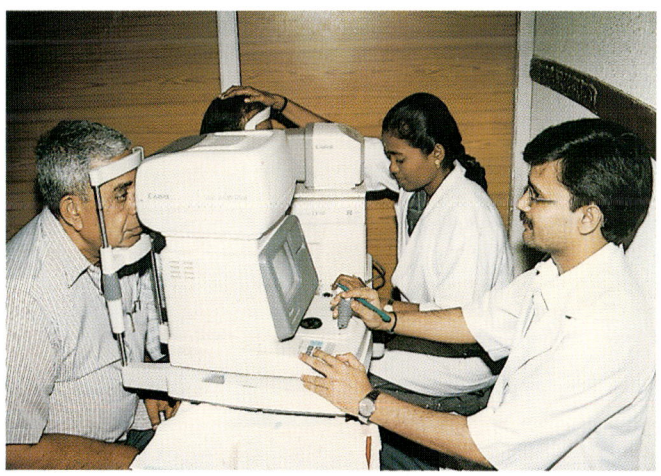

Figure 21: Auto-refractor. This machine does computerised eye testing. Next to the autorefractor is the non-contact tonometer which measures the Intraocular pressure of the eye.

Autorefractor. One should not have a prescription directly from the autorefractor, but use it to help give us a better reading of the power of the eye.

The Fundamental Principle of Eye Education and Relaxation

Do you read imperfectly? Do you notice then that when you look at the first word you do not see best where you are looking, that you might see other words just as well or better than the one you are looking at? Do you notice also that the harder you try to see the worse you see?

Now close your eyes and rest them, remembering some colour like black or white that you can remember perfectly. Keep the eyes closed until the feeling of strain has been completely relieved. Now open them and look at the first word of a sentence for a fraction of a second. If you have been able to relax, partially or completely, you will have a flash of improved or clear vision. Now close the eyes for a fraction of a second quickly, still remembering the colour and keep them closed till they feel rested. Then open them again for a fraction of a second. Continue this alternate resting of the eyes for a time and you may soon find that you can keep your eyes open longer than a fraction of a second without losing the improved vision.

If your trouble is with distant vision instead of near vision, use the same method with distant letters. In this way you can demonstrate to yourself the fundamental principle of eye education and relaxation.

Prevention of Defective Vision

The most important thing in preventing defective vision is to develop the habit of seeing without straining or without making any effort. This is done by learning how to use your eyes properly.

1. *Eyelids*

Nature has provided eyelids not only for the protection of the eyes from outside agencies, eg; dust, smoke etc., but also for the protection of our eyesight. When the upper eyelids remain lowered, the eye is at rest and the vision is better, but when the lids are raised the vision deteriorates. One should not squeeze the eyes and strain them while reading (Figs. 22 & 23).

2. *Blinking*

Blinking is a quick method of resting the eyes. Blinking is a natural habit of the eyes. In normal blinking, the upper eyelid comes down a little and is raised again. Blink once or twice while reading each line. The scientific reason why this is good is that whenever we blink the

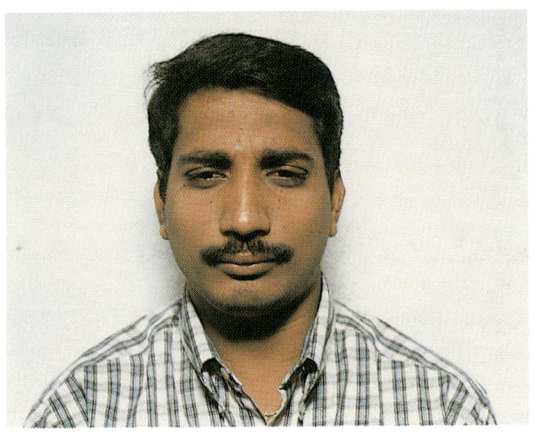

Figure 22: Person straining the eyes. This should not be done.

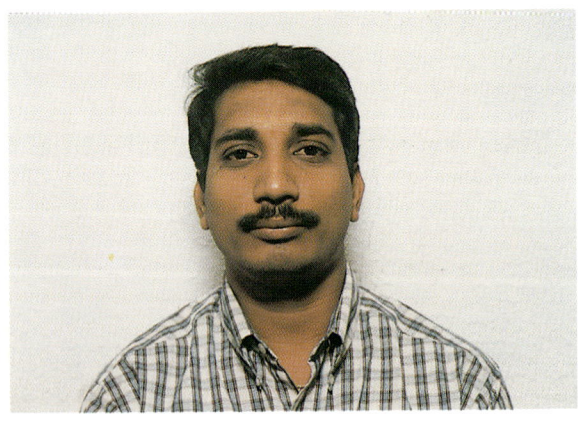

Figure 23: Person relaxed and not straining the eyes. This is the way one should look.

tear film of the eye flows past our cornea clearing it. This keeps our cornea moist and so refraction through the cornea is good.

3. Reading

While reading, keep the book at a lower level than the chin so that the lids are not raised. Move the head a little from side to side. Blink once or twice while reading each line. The distance of a book from the eyes should be where the print is seen at its best. It varies from individual to individual. Avoid reading in insufficiently illuminated places and in a lying posture. Keep the illumination of the light on the book.

4. *Writing*

While writing keep the sight on the point of the pen and move the sight with its movements. Blink frequently. A common mistake is to write forward and at the same time to look at the letters behind, which have already been written.

5. *Sewing*

Many women suffer from eye strain and headache while doing needle work. The common mistake is that they keep their eyes fixed on the cloth and blink only at very long intervals. They should move their sight with the movement of the needle and blink frequently (Figs. 24 & 25).

Television and the Eyes

Television has become firmly entrenched in our way of life. It keeps us uptodate on Wall street and World events. There are lots of questions one thinks about when one is watching television.

1. *Can Television Harm the Eyes?*

No. You cannot wear out your eyes by watching television. It does not cause eye defects. But if your child is watching television sitting very close to it, immediately consult an eye doctor(ophthalmologist) as the child might have a refractive error.

2. *How far should the Television be from us?*

The size of your television room and the television determine how far you should sit from the TV. A good general rule is: Stay as far from your TV screen as visual comfort permits.

3. *In what Position should we view the Picture?*

In order to see the picture without strain, sit comfortably by resting your back on the back of the chair. Keep the chin a little raised, the lids a little down and blink frequently (Fig.26).

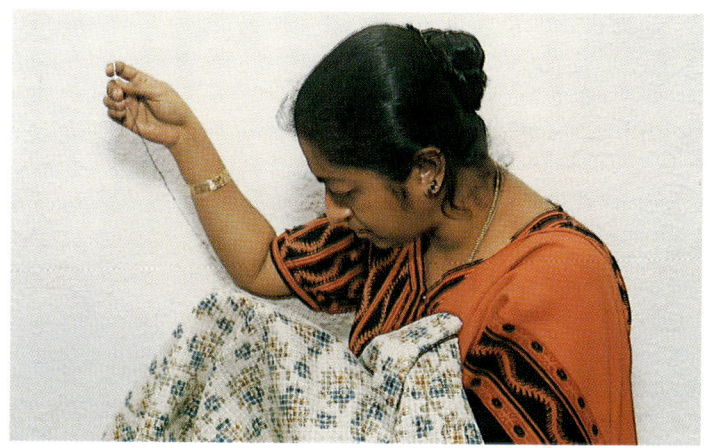

Figure 24: Sewing the wrong way. Note the eyes is still on the cloth and not on the needle, once the needle is out of the cloth.

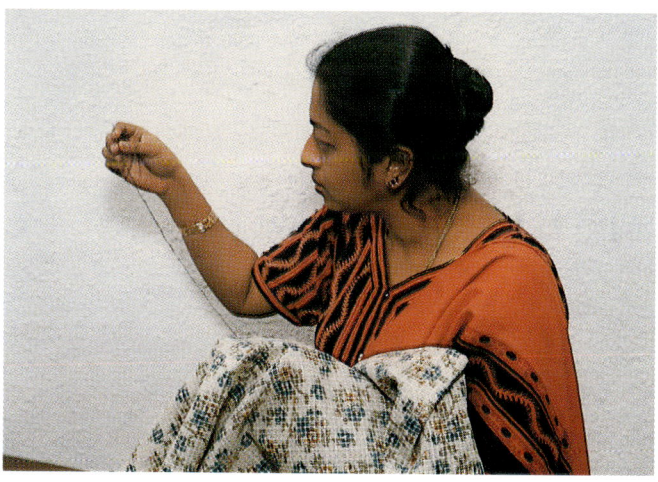

Figure 25: Sewing the right way. Note the eyes are always on the needle.

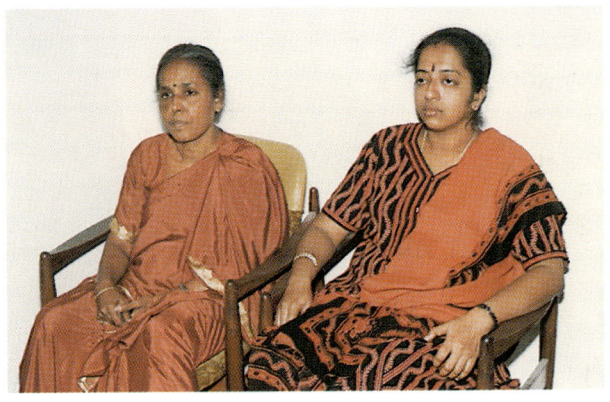

Figure 26: Method of watching TV. Don't be too close to the TV and keep at least one light in the room so that you do not strain the eyes while watching TV.

4. *Does Television involve Danger from X-Ray or other Radiation?*

No. There is no danger from radiation from TV screen.

5. *How should be the Room Lighting?*

One should have additional light in the viewing area or room. The contrast between the bright screen and surrounding darkness causes undue eye fatigue. Use soft, indirect lighting, making sure that no light source is reflected by the screen towards your eyes.

6. *Is a Large Screen better than Small Screen?*

In general, a large screen permits more comfortable viewing because it gives clearer vision at a greater distance. However a large screen in a small room is not recommended.

The Treatment of Defective Vision

Relaxation is one of the treatments of defective vision. Correct the position of the eyelids and eye ball. Exercises are very helpful. A good balanced and nourishing diet rich in proteins and vitamins help in the development of the eyes. Glasses and contact lenses are aids in correcting the vision.

Simple Exercises for Improving Vision

1. *Sun treatment*

Sit comfortably facing the sun with the eyes closed and sway the body gently from side to side like a pendulum for five minutes. **Remember to keep the eyes closed**. Hot sun at noon should be avoided. Morning or evening is the best time for sun treatment. It should be stopped as soon as the sun causes discomfort.

2. *Eye Wash*

After the sun treatment, come to the shade and wash the eyes with cold water.

3. *Palming*

Palming is a great relaxation for both the mind and the eyes. In palming, one should close and cover the eyes with the hollow of the palms, so as to shut off all light (Fig.27). Now a completely dark field will be observed before the eyes. After covering the eyes, imagine familiar things. This helps to relax the eyes. Do this for five minutes.

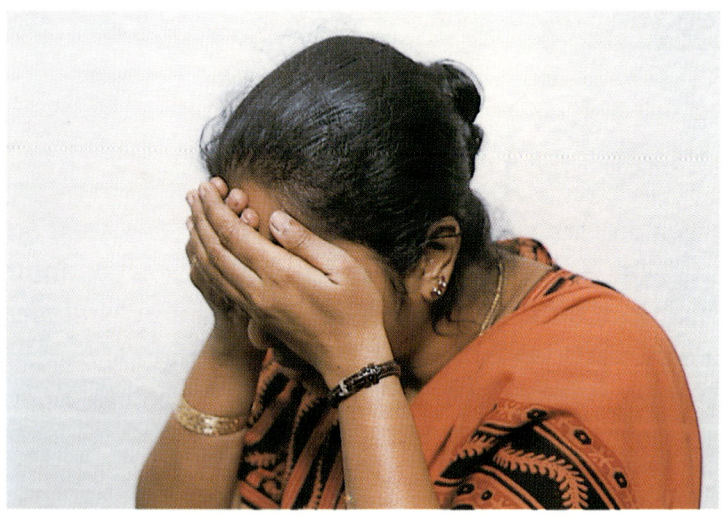

Figure 27: Palming. One should keep both the palms cupping the eyes and think of something one believes in. One should also keep the mind relaxed. A pillow can be placed under the elbows for more comfort.

4. *Central Fixation*

When the normal eye sees a thing, it sees only that part of the thing best on which it is fixed and other parts are not seen so well. This is called **Central Fixation**. Shift the sight from one line to another of the OM Chart (Fig. 28). Note that each line regarded separately appears best. While shifting the sight from one line to another, move the head along with the eyes. Blink at each corner.

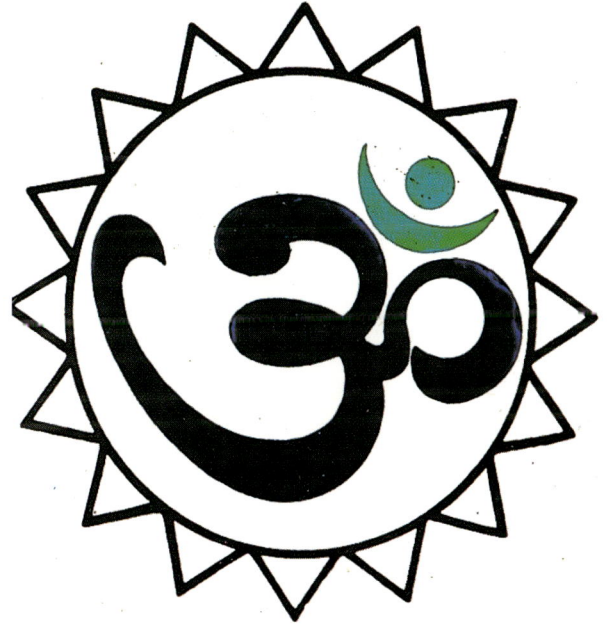

Figure 28: Om Chart.

5. *Fine-print Reading*

Fine-print reading at a distance where it is seen best is helpful in improving the vision. Blink once or twice in each line (Fig. 29).

Seven Truths of Normal Sight

1. Normal Sight can always be demonstrated in the normal eye, but only under favorable conditions.
2. Central Fixation: The letter or part of the letter regarded is always seen best.
3. Shifting: The point regarded changes rapidly and continuously.
4. Swinging: When the shifting is slow, the letters appear to move from side to side, or in other directions with a pendulum-like motion.
5. Memory is perfect. The color and background of the letters or other objects seen, are remembered perfectly, instantaneously and continuously.
6. Imagination is good. One may even see the white part of letters whiter than it really is, while the black is not altered by distance, illumination, size, or form of the letters.
7. Rest or relaxation of the eye and mind is perfect and can always be demonstrated.

When one of these seven fundamentals is perfect, all are perfect.

Figure 29: Fine-print reading.

6. *Fundamentals*

Read the Fundamentals with a card hole or glance at the white space in between the lines of the print. Blink once or twice in each line (Fig. 30).

Fundamentals
By W. H. Bates, M. D.

1. Central Fixation is seeing best where you are looking.

2. Favourable conditions: Light may be bright or dim. The distance of the print from the eyes, where seen best, also varies with people.

3. Shifting : With normal sight the eyes are moving all the time.

4. Swinging : When the eyes move slowly or rapidly from side to side, stationary objects appear to move in the opposite direction.

5. Long Swing : Stand with the feet about one foot apart, turn the body to the right—at the same time lifting the heel of the left foot. Do not move the head or eyes or pay any attention to the apparent movement of stationary objects. Now place the left heel on the floor, turn the body to the left, raising the heel of the right foot. Alternate.

6. Drifting Swing : When practising this swing, one pays no attention to the clearness of stationary objects, which appear to be moving. The eyes wander from point to point slowly, easily, or lazily, so that the stare or strain may be avoided.

7. Variable Swing: Hold the forefinger of one hand six inches from the right eye and about the same distance to the right, look straight ahead and move the head a short distance from side to side. The finger appears to move.

8. Stationary Objects Moving: By moving the head and eyes a short distance from side to side, being sure to blink, one can imagine stationary objects be moving.

9. Memory: Improving the memory of letters and other objects improves the vision for everything.

10. Imagination: We see only what we think we see, or what we imagine. We can only imagine what we remember.

11. Rest: All cases of imperfect sight are improved by closing the eyes and resting them.

12. Palming: The closed eyes may be covered with the palm of one or both hands.

13. Blinking: The normal eye blinks or closes and opens very frequently.

14. Mental Pictures: As long as one is awake one has all kinds of memories of mental pictures. If these are remembered easily, perfectly, the vision is benefited.

Figure 30: Fundamentals.

Contact Lenses

What are Contact Lenses?

Contact lenses are small, thin plastic discs that are designed to rest on the transparent window of the eye called the cornea (Figs. 31 and 32). The cornea is the clear front surface of the eye (Figs. 2 and 3). There are three types of contact lenses: **Hard**, **Semi-soft** and **Soft**. Hard lenses are sometimes called "rigid" lenses, semi-soft "gas-permeable" and soft lenses "flexible" lenses.

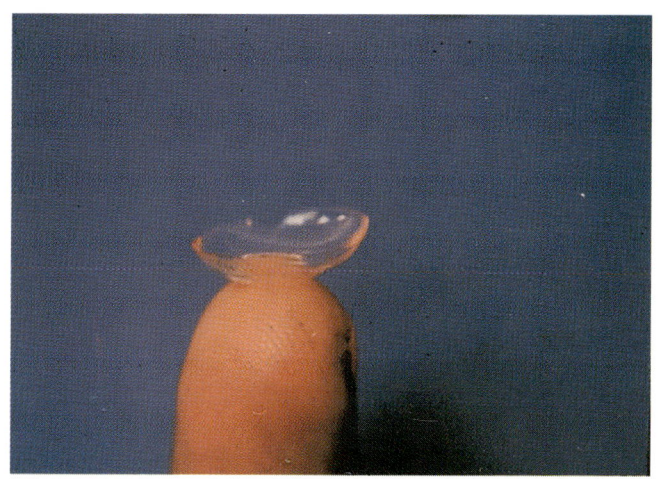

Figure 31: Contact lens. Note how small the contact lens is.

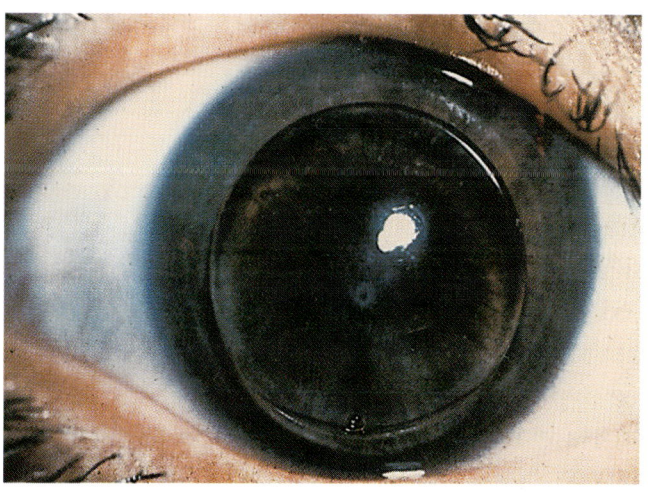

Figure 32: Contact lens fitting on the cornea.

What are they used for?

Contact lenses are used to correct refractive errors. They are also used to correct certain special eye diseases. Normally, the cornea is spherical. If a patient has a cornea which is conical then the condition is called a **Conical Cornea** or **Keratoconus**. In such a condition contact lenses are given so that the pressure of the contact lens on the cornea flattens it. If a patient has a white mark on the cornea then also coloured contact lenses can be given for cosmetic reasons so that the white opacity is not seen. Film stars can use coloured contact lenses while acting, to change the colour of their eyes.

What are the advantages of contact lenses over spectacles?

Contact lenses are cosmetically very good as the patient does not wear glasses. Further, the side vision is better. Contact lenses should be used if the difference in power of the two eyes is more than 5 Dioptres, as if glasses are prescribed for such a patient the patient will start seeing double. This is because the two eyes cannot cope with a difference of more than 5 Dioptres with glasses but this can be done with contact lenses. Contact lenses give a more normal sized image than spectacles. Contact lenses are also preferred in refractive errors of high degrees.

Lens Insertion and Care

It is very easy to insert and remove a contact lens. The procedure is taught to the patient by a contact lens specialist and it takes about a week to learn. Lens care is also not a bother. It is a responsibility. It requires a few minutes each day of good hygiene and good habits. In a nutshell, it is cleaning, rinsing and disinfecting your lenses. If one keeps the lenses clean, there are generally no risks. The problems that can occur are a scratch on the eye or an eye infection. These occur very rarely.

Zyoptix Laser/Lasik Laser

LASIK is short for 'Laser-assisted *in-situ* Keratomileusis'. The basic idea in Lasik is to get the patient's dependency on glasses removed. For this treatment with an **Excimer Laser** is done on the front window of the eye called the cornea (Figs. 2 and 3). The cornea has five layers, namely

A. A(E)pithelium
B. Bowman's Membrane
C. Connective Tissue

D. Descemet's Membrane and
E. Endothelium

For any treatment to remove the refractive error of the eye the **Excimer Laser Ablation** has to be done on the middle layer which is layer C or the connective tissue of the cornea. The idea is to make the central cornea thinner in myopic patients and thicker in hypermetropic patients, thus reducing their glass power.

Excimer Photorefractive Keratectomy (PRK)

The old technology was the PRK, otherwise known as the **Photorefractive Keratectomy Treatment**. In this the Excimer laser is applied onto layers A, then layer B, and finally layer C. The disadvantage of this is that when layer A gets damaged the patient has pain and when layer B gets damaged the patient will have scar formation in the cornea.

Lasik Laser

Dr Ioannis Pallikaris from Greece started a technique called Lasik in which layers A and B are first cut with a special instrument called a **Microkeratome** and flapped back (Figs. 33 and 34). Then the Excimer laser is applied

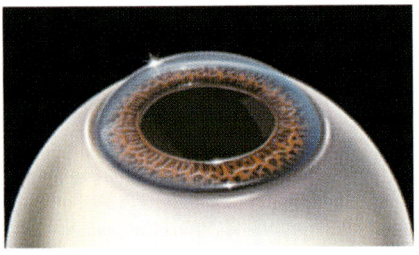

Figure 33: Cornea with normal curvature.

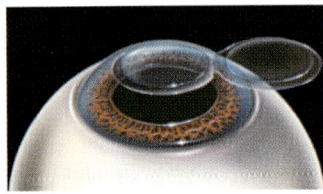

Figure 34: Cornea with flap open. The flaps of layer A and B are made by a special instrument called the microkeratome.
(Fig 33 to 43 *Courtesy*: Dr Jerry Tan, Singapore)

directly on layer C (Fig. 35). In myopic patients this laser application is done on the central portion of the cornea making it thin. Once the laser ablation is completed the flap of layer A and B are then placed back onto the cornea (Fig. 36). The advantage of this is that layers A and B are not damaged and so the patient does not have any pain or discomfort. Scarring is also avoided as layer B is not damaged. Thus a myopic or short-

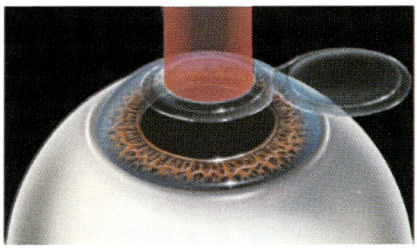

Figure 35: Excimer laser application (seen in red) is applied on to the central portion of the cornea on to layer C. This makes the central portion of the cornea thin to correct short sight (myopia).

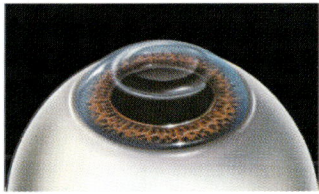

Figure 36: Flap is replaced back in position once the laser ablation is completed.

sighted patient (Fig. 37) can see well after Lasik laser as the cornea has been flattened (Fig. 38).

In hypermetropia or long sight (Fig 39) the flap is first created and then the laser is applied onto the periphery of the cornea (Fig. 40) thus making the periphery thin and the central portion of the cornea thick. The flap is then replaced back in position (Fig. 41). Thus a hypermetropic or long-sighted patient (Fig. 42)

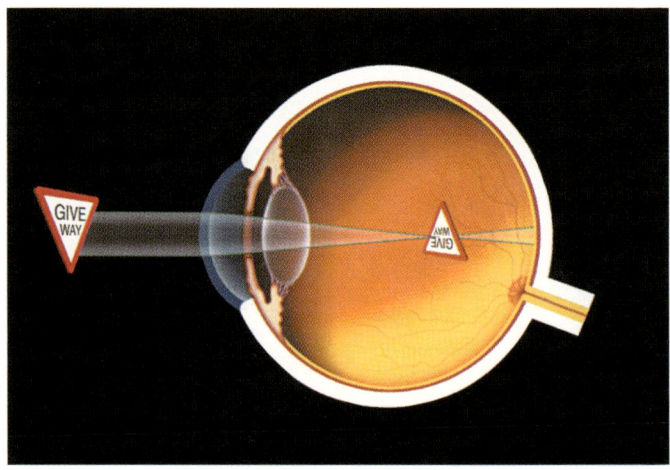

Figure 37: Myopic patient. The image is focused in front of the retina.

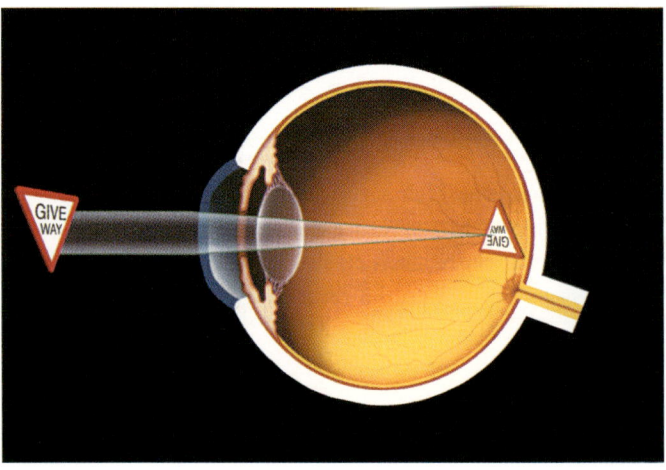

Figure 38: After Lasik Laser. The image is now focused on to the retina. This happens because the cornea has been flattened.

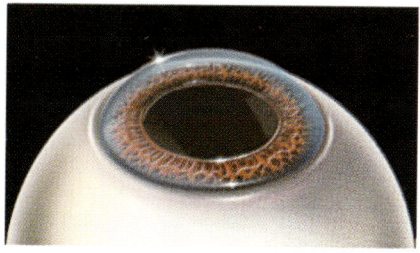

Figure 39: Hypermetropic eye.

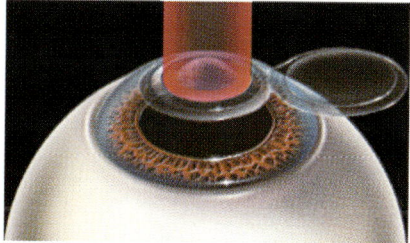

Figure 40: Cornea cut and flap made. Excimer laser is done on the periphery of the cornea so that the periphery of the cornea becomes thin. This makes the central cornea thicker in comparision correcting long sight (hypermetropia).

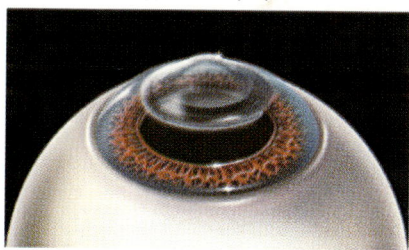

Figure 41: Flap of cornea replaced back in position. Note the central thickness of the cornea corrects the hypermetropia.

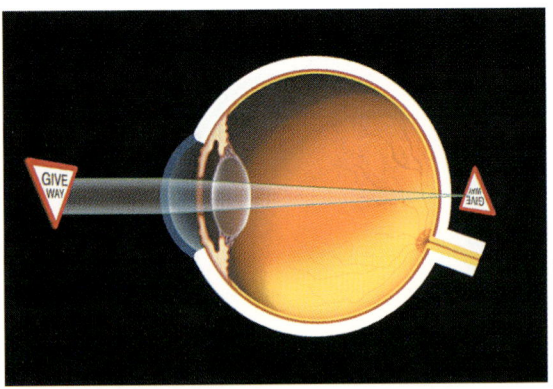

Figure 42: Hypermetropic patient. The image is focused behind the retina.

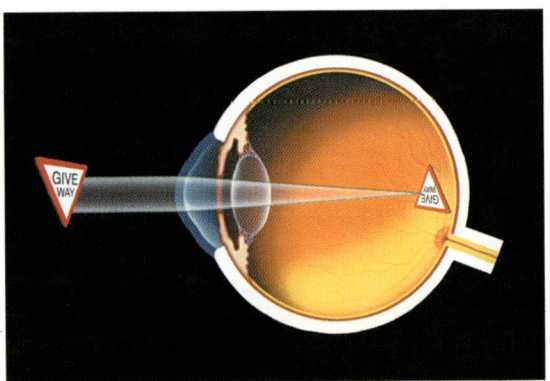

Figure 43: After Lasik Laser. The image is now focused on to the retina. This happens because the cornea has been made thin in the periphery and the central portion is thick.

can see well after Lasik laser as the cornea has been made thin in the periphery and thicker in the centre (Fig. 43).

The whole treatment takes about 10 minutes. There is no injection, no stitches and no pad placed after the Laser treatment. Both eyes are generally done simultaneously. The **Zyoptix/Lasik Laser machine** (Fig. 44) is a very delicate machine and is kept in a room which has to have 20 degrees Centigrade temperature and 50 % humidity.

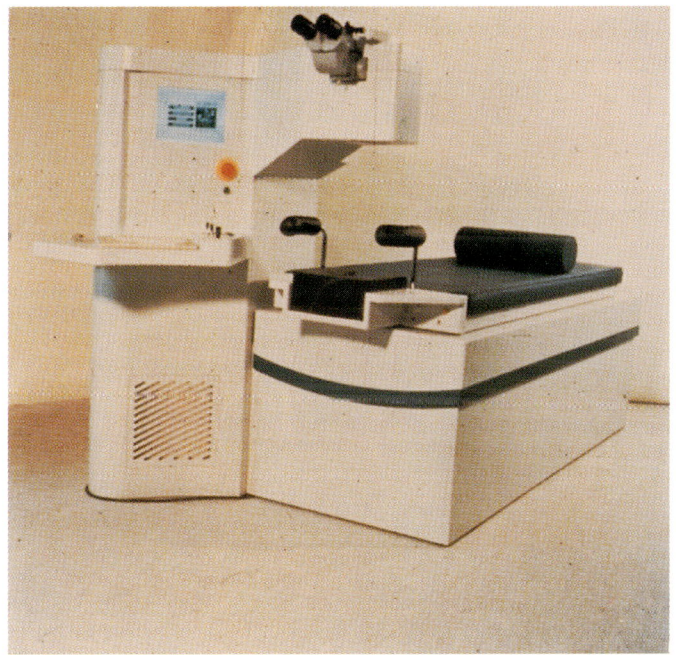

Figure 44: Zyoptix Lasik Laser Machine.

Zyoptix Laser

The latest machine for advanced eye care treatment is the **Zyoptix Laser**. (Fig. 44), made by Bausch and Lomb. It is a machine to give personalised correction so that patients achieve better quality of vision.

Every person has got in his or her eye aberrations. This creates a problem for vision. Today, a new discovery and invention is the **Wavefront Technology**. In this a special machine called an **Aberrometer** (Fig. 45) is used. This takes images from the patients eye and analyses the aberrations present. Then the patient is

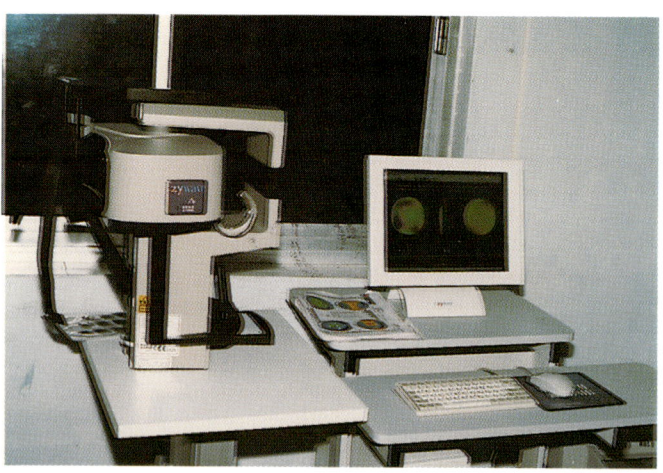

Figure 45: Aberrometer machine which checks the aberrations present in the eye. This machine also detects the new refractive error called Aberropia.

put on another machine called the **Orbscan** (Fig. 46). Once the data from these two machines are obtained the doctor is able to analyse the extent of aberrations and defect of the eye.

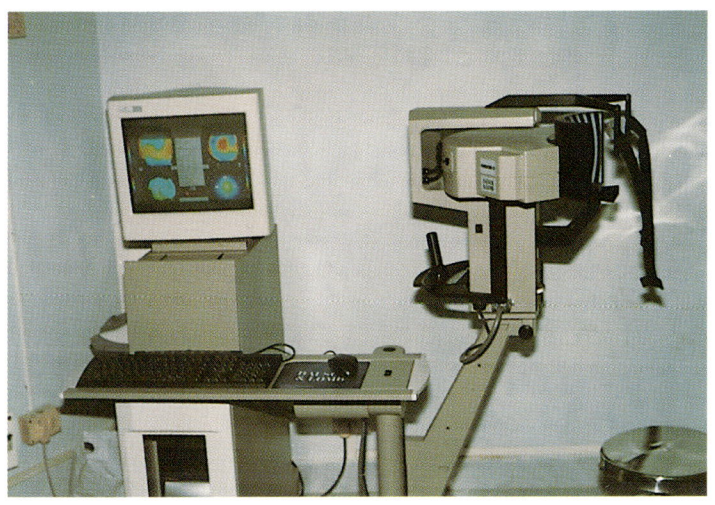

Figure 46: Orbscan machine. This is a corneal topography machine which analyses the cornea thoroughly for any abnormality before the lasik procedure.

Then these data are linked on to the Zyoptix Laser. The laser then ablates the cornea. In other words, laser is done on the middle layers of the cornea. The amount of treatment done on the cornea depends upon the input received from the aberrometer and orbscan. This link to the Zyoptix Laser is crucial. The laser then removes not only the patient's myopia or hypermetropia but also removes all the aberrations in the eye. This gives the patient a better vision and result.

This sort of custom ablation, which means for each person a special laser application, helps the patient tremendously. This is because it is an individualised treatment for each patient. Patients achieve better vision with the Zyoptix Laser than with ordinary Lasik Laser which is not a personalised laser treatment for each patient.

The whole treatment takes about 15-20 minutes for both eyes. There is no injection, no pad, no stitches and no hospitalisation. The next day the patient can go back to his or her routine work.

Headache

One of the most common complaints of an eye patient is headache. While the majority of cases complaining of headache are due to eye trouble and strain, some are due to overeating, constipation, cold, ill-health, high blood pressure, sinus troubles and brain affection for which a physician should be consulted.

In most cases headache is due to wrong use of the eyes while reading, writing, watching movies etc. Correcting the habit of seeing is the cure for it. Many times the headache is due to mental strain. Such cases are helped by palming (Fig. 27) and fine print reading (Fig. 29).

Some people get headache after putting on glasses. It may be that either the power of the glass is not correct or the lenses have not been fitted properly. Consult an eye doctor for proper prescription of glasses.

Severe headache and eye pain especially after sleep may be due to glaucoma which indicates an increased pressure on the eyes. This is a serious problem and needs immediate attention.

Most of the time the headache is due to defective vision. Exercises and glasses for improving vision help to relieve the headache.

Red Eye

A red eye is a common condition which most of us have developed at some time or the other. This is generally due to an infection which we have developed by a germ entering the eye through the air. The eyes are painful and watery. Some whitish material will be coming out of the eyes continuously (Fig. 47).This condition is called **Conjunctivitis** which means an infection of the conjunctiva (Fig. 2 and 3). The treatment of this is to wash the eyes with cold water. Use an antibiotic eye drop in the eye. Do not

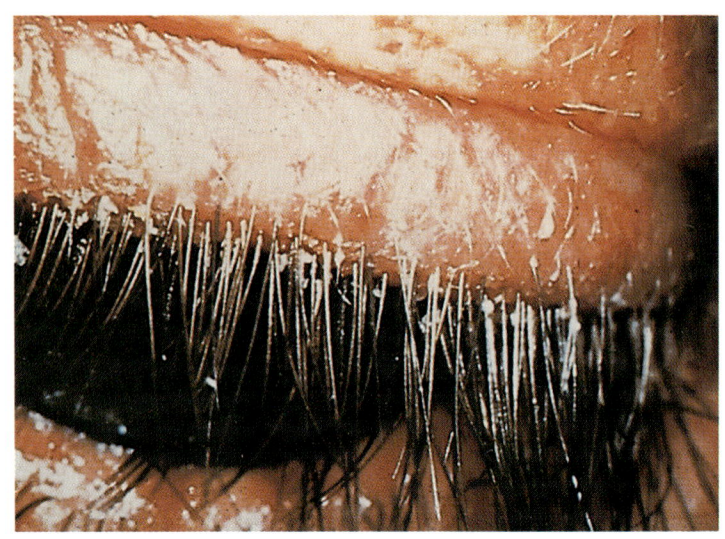

Figure 47: Conjunctivitis. Note the lids are matted with discharge. The patient should be put on antibiotic eye drops and keep good ocular hygiene. One should see that one does not meet too many people at this time so that the conjunctivitis does not spread to others.

apply any home-made remedies. It is best to consult an eye doctor as soon as possible.

Though Conjunctivitis is the most common cause of a red eye, there are other causes also. An infection of the inside of the eye, glaucoma or injury to the eye can also cause a red eye. A serious infection of one week's duration is likely to cause permanent damage to the eyes so one should not ignore it and consult an eye doctor.

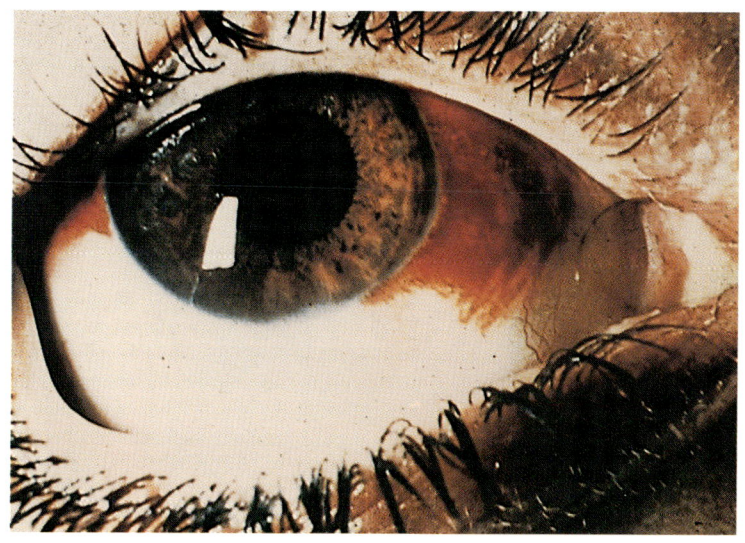

Figure 48: Subconjunctival haemorrhage. Note the red area from the blood clot. This will gradually absorb and become all right in a couple of weeks.

Another cause of a red eye is an injury to the eye. This can produce a bleed in the conjunctival area and is called a **Subconjunctival haemorrhage** (Fig. 48). This is by and large not dangerous as it is absorbed in a couple of weeks, but one should check with an eye doctor to see if there is any other bleed inside the eye.

Some patients develop a boil in the lids (Fig. 49). This is called a **Chalazion**. This needs treatment with antibiotic drops and hot formentation. In hot formentation, one

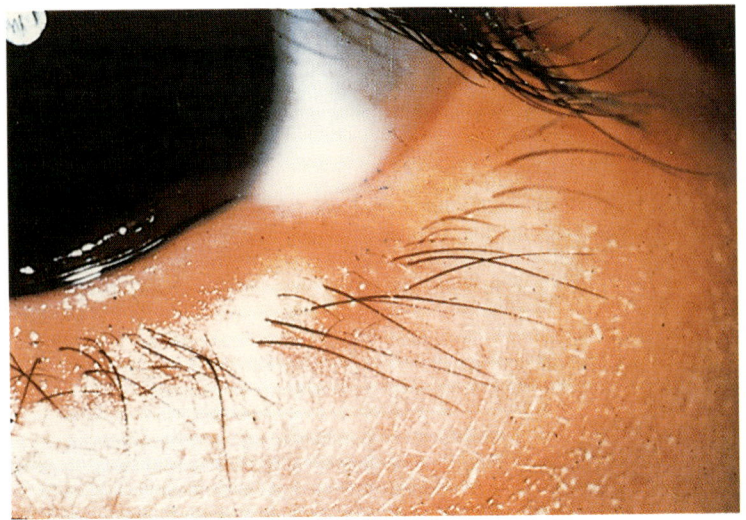

Figure 49: Chalazion. In the lower lid there is a boil. This needs treatment with antibiotic eye drops and fomentation. If it does not become all right the eye doctor might have to incise it and clear it. One should also check for any refractive power in such cases.

should take a handkerchief and place it on a hot iron box. Once the kerchief becomes warm, one should close the eye and apply it on the chalazion area. If it does not become all right within a week one should go to an eye doctor who will incise (cut) it and clear it.

Cataract

What is Cataract?

Cataract is an opacity in the lens of the eye (Fig. 50). In a camera, an object is focused on the film by a lens (Fig.1). Similarly, an object seen by the eye is focused on the retina by its lens. When the lens of our eye gets opaque, it is called **Cataract**. The normal lens allows light to reach the retina. When it becomes opaque and does not allow light to reach the retina, we are unable to see clearly.

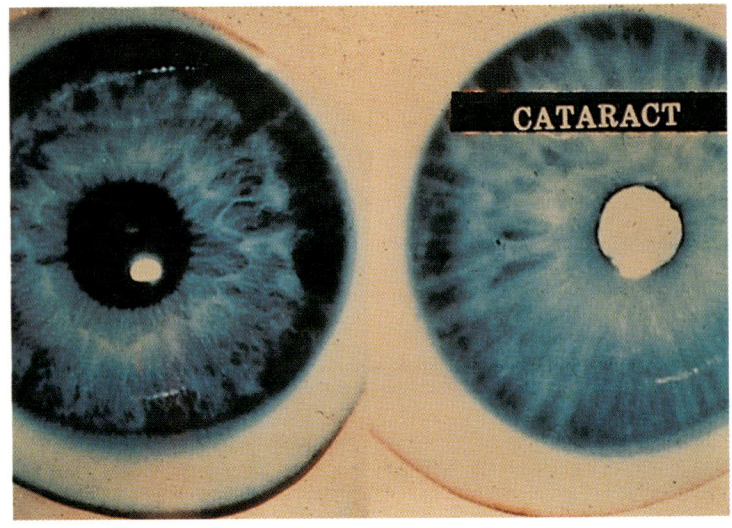

Figure 50: Cataract. The figure on the left is that of a normal eye and that on the right of a patient with cataract. Note the white opacity in the centre which is the cataract. This opacity is in the lens of the eye.

To understand cataract better, imagine photographing through a camera with grease smeared on its lens (Fig. 51). In such a case, the image formed is very hazy and blurred. Similar to grease smearing on the lens of a camera, if the lens of the eye gets opaque, the image formed on the retina will be blurred and one will not see clearly.

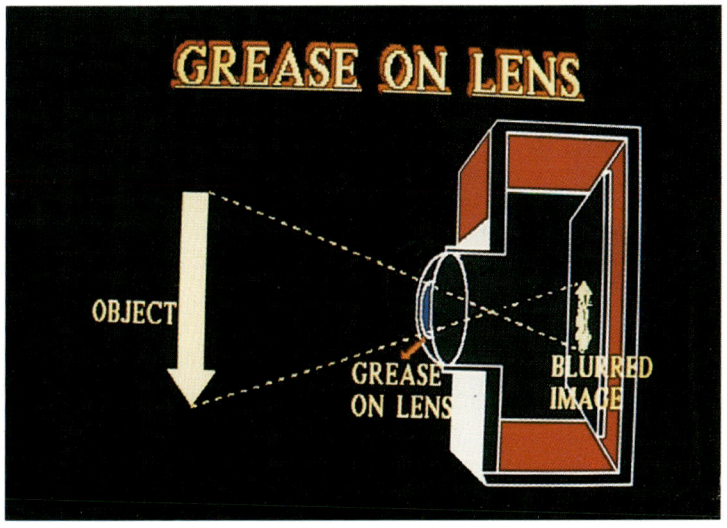

Figure 51: Grease on a camera lens is akin to an opacity in the lens of the eye. Just as grease on the lens of a camera makes the image blurred, an opacity in the lens of the eye makes the image blurred for the patient as light is not able to travel properly through the lens to reach the retina.

History of Cataract Surgery

The history of cataract dates back to 3000 years. The earliest cataract operation was performed by the famous surgeon of ancient India, Susruta, a disciple of Danavantri. Even in that ancient era, Susruta described cataract as an opacity of the lens. He has given an admirable account of the technique of its treatment by couching which he successfully practised. In this operation he displaced the opaque cataract-affected lens away from the centre of the eye to another part of the eye. Today modern medical advances have made cataract surgery one of the most successful forms of surgery. New surgical techniques and Intraocular lenses can restore excellent vision in 97% of the cases. In the 1960s Dr Charles Kelman from USA started a technique called **Phacoemulsification** in which cataracts were removed through a 3 mm incision, compared to a 12 mm incision in which the whole cataract was removed in toto. Then in 1998, Dr Amar Agarwal from India started a technique called **Phakonit** in which cataracts were removed through a 0.9 mm opening. In the year 2001 a special lens was made which went through this small opening of 1 to 1.5 mm. This was called the **Rollable Intraocular lens**. The technique of no anesthesia cataract surgery was also started by Dr Amar Agarwal of India.

Why does Cataract Form?

The causes of the formation of cataract are not fully known. It is basically an ageing phenomenon. Just as our hair gets grey, so also does the lens of our eye get opaque. Next to old age come other factors like deficency of food like proteins and vitamins, some toxic drugs, general diseases like diabetes, infections and injuries. Sometimes German measles in pregnant mothers causes cataract in the child.

Tips Beneficial to Delay the Onset of Cataract

1. Take good and nourishing diet rich in proteins and vitamins. Food such as liver, eggs, milk products, carrots, cabbages and yeast are good.
2. Protect your eyes from excessive exposure to sun's rays, X-rays, intense heat and injuries.
3. Diseases such as diabetes and syphillis should be treated early and effectively.

Treatment of Cataract

There is no medical treatment for cataract. The only treatment is surgery. The important question is when should one get operated for cataract. This depends on the occupation of the patient. If the patient is a pilot, he should be operated immediately, for even a slight deterioration of vision will affect his work, whereas if the patient is a housewife, she can delay surgery for some time. When a person has cataract and the decision is made to operate, then the diseased lens is removed and replaced by an artificial lens.

Alternatives to the Natural Lens

Once the cataract (diseased lens) is removed, there is no focusing ability of the eye as there is no lens in the eye. So one has to use an artificial lens to get the object focused on the retina. This can be either in the form of a spectacle, contact lens or an Intraocular lens.

1. Spectacles can be used but these are heavy and not comfortable. Further, if one removes these glasses the person is blind. Other disadvantages of these glasses is that everything is magnified and the side view is very poor.
2. The second alternative is to use a contact lens. This is an artificial lens placed on the eye (Figs.31 and 32). The disadvantage of this as with spectacles is that if we remove it the person is blind as there is no focusing ability. Another problem with contact lenses is that they have to be put on in the morning and removed at night, which is difficult for an old person.
3. So, the best method is to give the patient an **Intraocular lens**. This is an artificial lens that is placed in the eye at the time of surgery. It will remain in place till the end of life. By this all the problems of spectacles or contact lenses is removed. This lens does not irritate the eye. Specialised instruments

are used prior to the surgery to assess the patient. An **Ultrascan** is used to get the view of the inside of the eye (Fig. 52). A **Biometer** is used to calculate the power of the Intraocular lens to be implanted in the eye (Fig. 53).

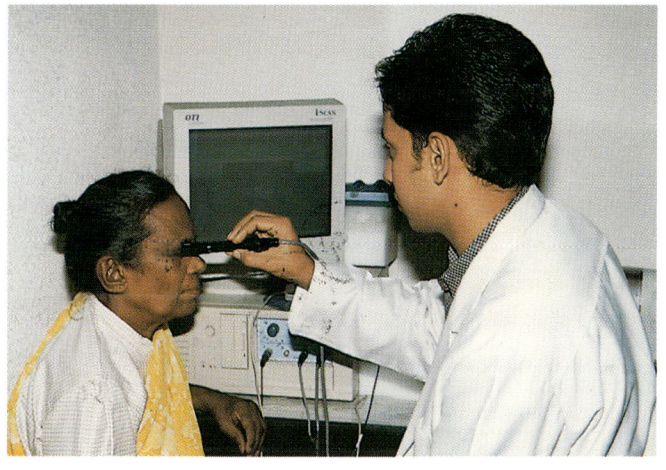

Figure 52: Ultrascan. This gives the details of the inside of the eye.

Out-patient Cataract Surgery

Today, we are able to operate patients with cataract and remove their defective lens and replace it with an artificial lens called an Intraocular lens as an out-patient procedure. The patient comes in the morning for

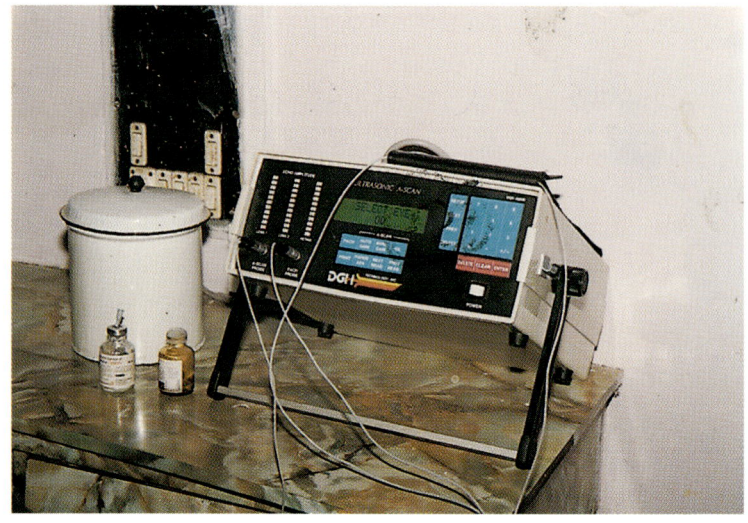

Figure 53: Biometer. This calculates the Intraocular lens power one should implant in the patient.

surgery and after the operation can go home. The surgery is done without any injection, without any pad and without any stitch being placed in the eye.

This is called the no injection, no pad, no stitch cataract surgical technique.

The patients are not admitted in the hospital. They come in the morning and can go back after the cataract removal and the **IOL** fixed in their eye. The patients can go back to work the next day.

Manual Cataract Extraction Technique

The manual or the old technique for cataract removal uses a 12 mm incision (cut) to remove the cataract. One technique called the **Intracapsular Cataract Extraction** (Fig. 54) has an incision of 12 mm. In this the entire cataract is removed with the capsule of the lens. The disadvantage of this technique is that the artificial lens called the Intraocular lens (IOL) is placed in the anterior chamber. As there is no capsule the IOL cannot be placed in the capsular bag.

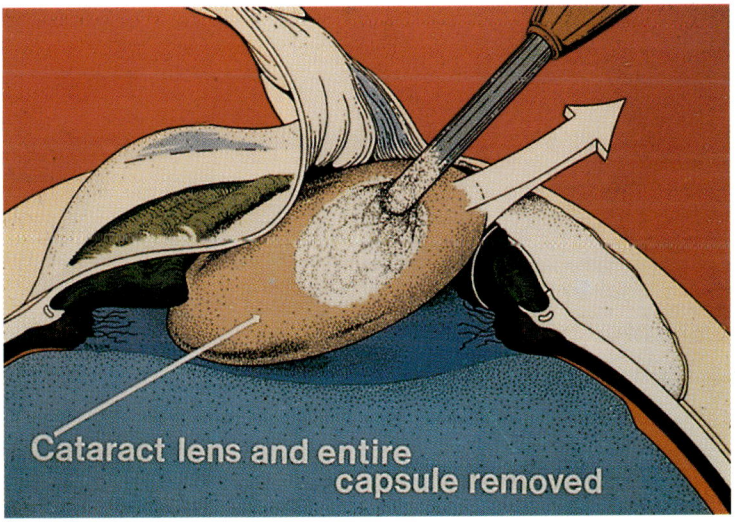

Figure 54: Intracapsular cataract extraction. In this the cataract affected lens is removed with the capsule of the lens.

Another manual technique is called the **Extracapsular Cataract Extraction Technique** (Fig. 55). In this the incision is about 10-12 mm. In this the cataract is removed but the capsule of the lens is left behind. The advantage of this technique is that the artificial lens called the Intraocular lens (IOL) is placed in the capsular bag with the capsule of the lens acting as a support for the lens. The disadvantage of this technique is that

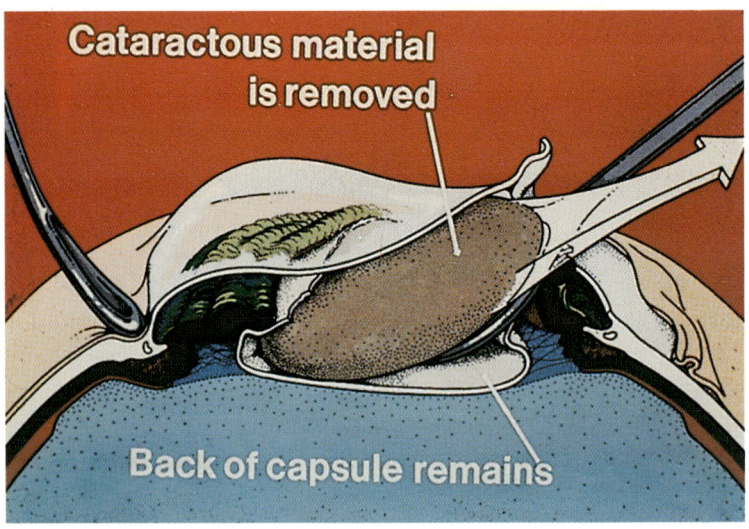

Figure 55: Extracapsular cataract extraction. In this the cataract affected lens is removed and the capsule of the lens is left behind. The advantage of this is that normally the artifical lens or intra-ocular lens which has to be placed in the eye is placed on the capsule for support. As the capsule is still present an Intraocular lens can be placed in the original position of the lens. The disadvantage of this technique is that the incision is too large and is about 10-12 mm.

the incision is quite large, of about 10-12 mm, which creates scarring in the eye. This means half the eye is cut open and then an IOL is inserted inside the eye. The IOL is about 6 mm and so easily goes inside the eye. Sutures are then placed and the patient admitted. The patient takes rest for 45 days and after that suitable glasses are prescribed. The patient is given spectacles for fine tuning after 45 days.

Phacoemulsification

Dr Charles Kelman from USA started a technique called Phacoemulsification in the 60s to remove cataract through a 3 mm opening. Since then various new modalities have developed which have made this technique more refined. The machine for removing the cataracts is called a **Phacoemulsifier machine** (Fig. 56) which cuts the cataract into small pieces and removes them by aspiration.

The first step in Phacoemulsification is to make an incision (Fig. 57) of 3 mm. Note that in the figure the right hand has a diamond knife which makes the incision of 3 mm. The left hand holds a rod to stabilise the eye. Then after the front capsule of the lens is removed the Phacoemulsification probe is held in the right hand and a chopping instrument in the left hand (Fig. 58). The

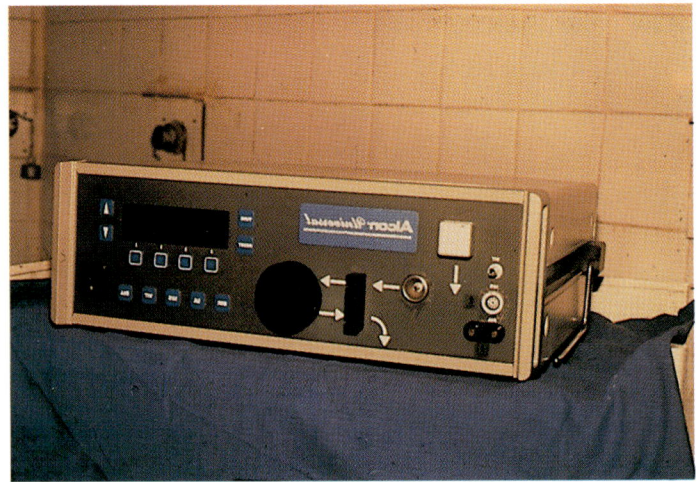

Figure 56: Phacoemulsifier machine.

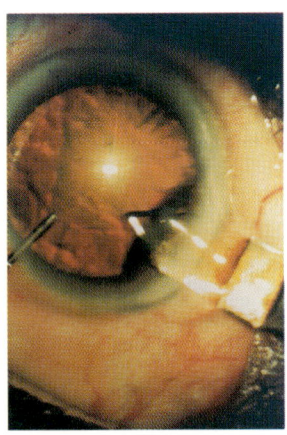

Figure 57: Phacoemulsification technique. The first step is to make the incision of 3 mm with the right hand. This is done with a special diamond knife.

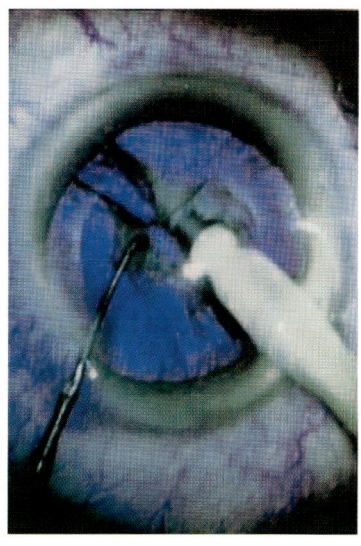

Figure 58: Phacoemulsification technique.
The phacoemulsification probe now is held in the right hand with a chopper in the left hand and this chops the cataract into small pieces which are then aspirated and removed out of the eye through the 3 mm opening.

Phacoemulsification probe and the chopper help to cut the defective lens into small pieces and finally remove the entire lens through the 3 mm opening (Fig. 59). Note that the cataract has been totally removed. Then a special lens called a **Foldable Intraocular lens** is taken and inserted inside the eye (Fig. 60). This is done with a special injecting system. Once the lens is fully in the capsular bag (Fig. 61) one can see the lens filling the whole space of the capsular bag.

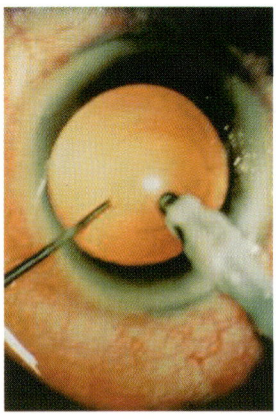

Figure 59: Phacoemulsification technique. The cataract has been totally removed.

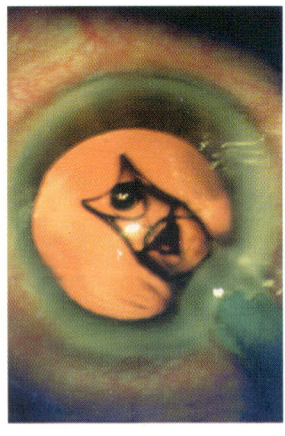

Figure 60: Phacoemulsification technique. The foldable Intraocular lens is inserted inside the eye with a special injector.

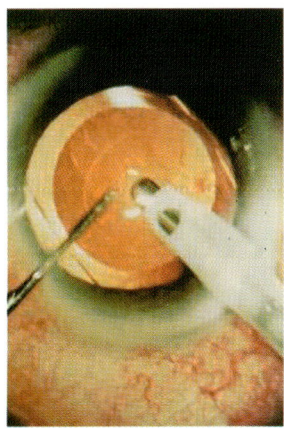

Figure 61: Phacoemulsification technique. The foldable Intraocular lens has unfolded and is lying on the capsule of the lens.

Foldable Intraocular Lenses

Normally, lenses used are rigid and cannot be folded. The problem of this is that one has to make a large cut or incision in the eye to implant these lenses. Today, the latest development in Intraocular lenses is the Foldable Intraocular lens. These are special lenses which come from USA. These can be folded. Once they are folded they are placed in a special cartridge and then the cartridge is placed in a special injector. The injector is passed into the eye and the lens is also gradually passed into the eye. The lens unfolds in the eye. These lenses can be passed into the eye through a very small cut. Thus this foldable Intraocular lens helps make the incision very small.

Putting large lenses in large incisions is bucking the tide of history. Small incisions offer the best chance for the most rapid, stable visual rehabilitation of the cataract patient at the least cost, including the time of impaired vision following surgery, the need for follow up care, the attendance of relatives to take care of the patient and the like.

The advantages of using a foldable Intraocular lens due to the very small size of the cut made in the eye are:

1. The patient is not admitted in the hospital.
2. The patient comes for the surgery and goes back immediately after a few hours in the hospital.
3. There are no stitches.
4. The patient gets back to his or her normal routine the next day and can go to office, have a full bath or do normal housework like cooking, etc.

Phakonit

One of the biggest breakthroughs in cataract removal has come from Dr Agarwal's Eye Hospital. This is called Phakonit. In this the 1 mm barrier to remove cataracts has been broken.

On 15 August 1998 at Dr Agarwal's Eye Hospital, Dr Amar Agarwal performed the first sub-1 mm cataract surgery by a technique called Phakonit. In this the cataract was removed through a 0.9 mm incision. This technique is absolutely painless and the patient does not require any injection at all. Since the incision is below 1 mm the patient has no injection, no stitches and no pad. The patient walks inside the hospital and goes back immediately. The duration of treatment is between 5 and 10 minutes.

The first step is to make an incision of 0.9 mm (Fig. 62). This is done with a special knife. Then the instruments for Phakonit are passed into the eye (Fig. 63)

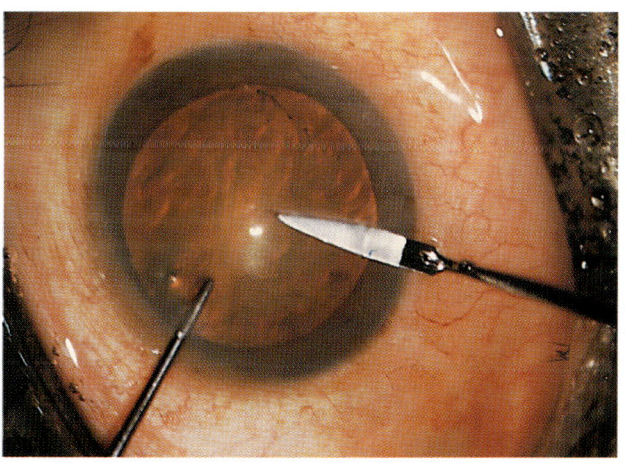

Figure 62: Phakonit technique. An incision of 0.9 mm is first made.

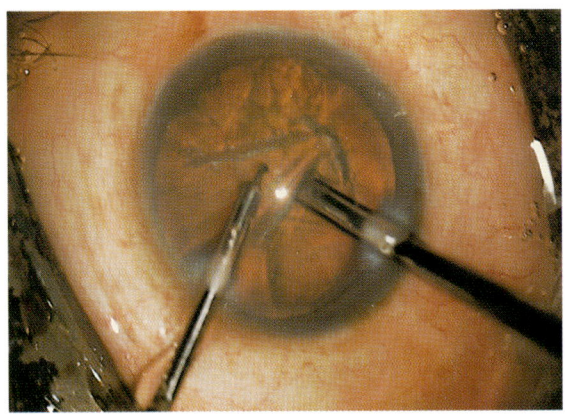

Figure 63: Phakonit technique. The instruments of phakonit are passed into the eye.

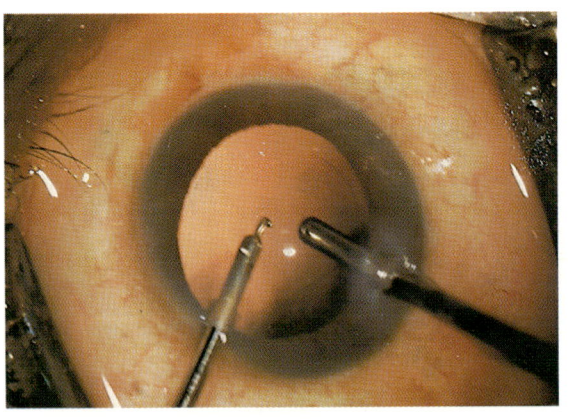

Figure 64: Phakonit technique. The whole cataract has been removed by cutting it into small pieces and aspirating it.

and the cataract cut into small pieces by Phakonit (Fig. 64) and finally the whole cataract is removed.

The problem with this technique was to find an IOL which would pass through such a small incision. Then on 2 October 2001 the first case of a 5 mm Optic Phakonit Rollable IOL was done by Dr Amar Agarwal. This was done in their Chennai (India) hospital. The lens used was a special lens from USA (Fig. 65). This was the first Rollable IOL which was implanted after a Phakonit procedure and as it was a rolled IOL. It has been called "**Phakonit Rollable IOL**".

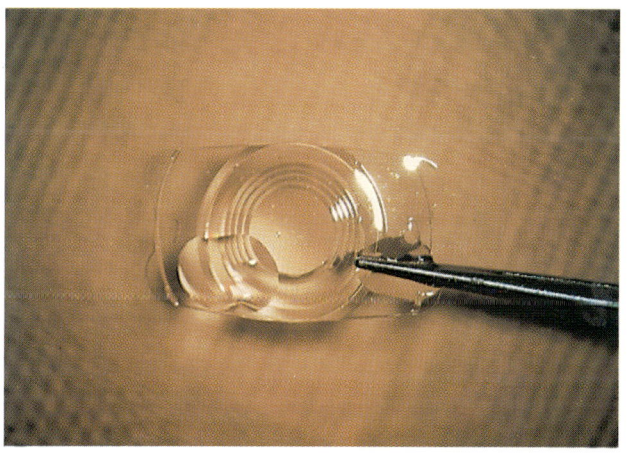

Figure 65: Rollable IOL implantation technique.
The rollable IOL held with forceps.

The advantage of this lens is that it is a very thin lens and when placed in water becomes pliable and can

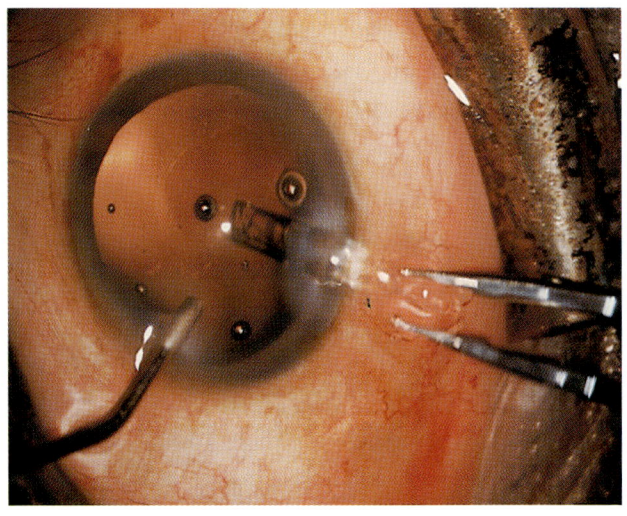

Figure 66: Rollable IOL implantation technique. The rollable IOL is rolled and inserted into the eye.

then be rolled and inserted into the eye (Fig. 66). Inside the eye the lens opens gradually (Fig. 67). The patient can come to the hospital and go home immediately. The advantages are that the incision now has become very small.

Acritec IOL

Another lens can be implanted in the eye through a 1.5 mm incision. This is the **Acritec Intraocular lens (IOL)**. This lens is a special foldable IOL that can pass

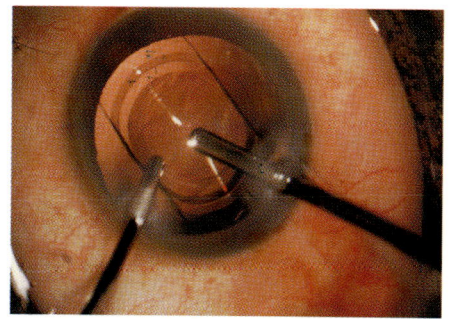

Figure 67: Rollable IOL implantation technique. The rollable IOL has unrolled and is in the capsular bag.

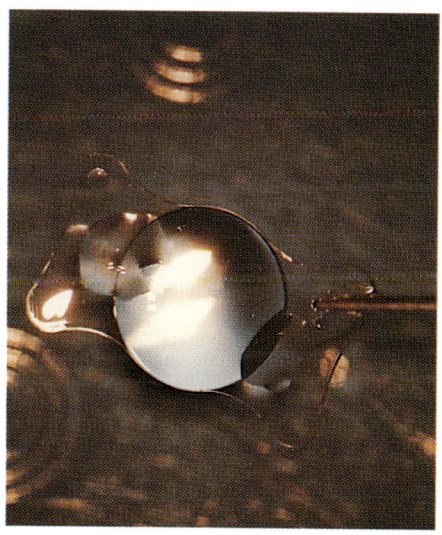

Figure 68: Acritec IOL implantation technique. The acritec IOL is a special foldable IOL that passes through a 1.5 mm incision. The lens is held with forceps.

through a 1.5 mm incision (Fig 68). The lens is then loaded on to an injector and injected inside the eye (Fig 69). Once inside the eye the lens unfolds (Fig 70).

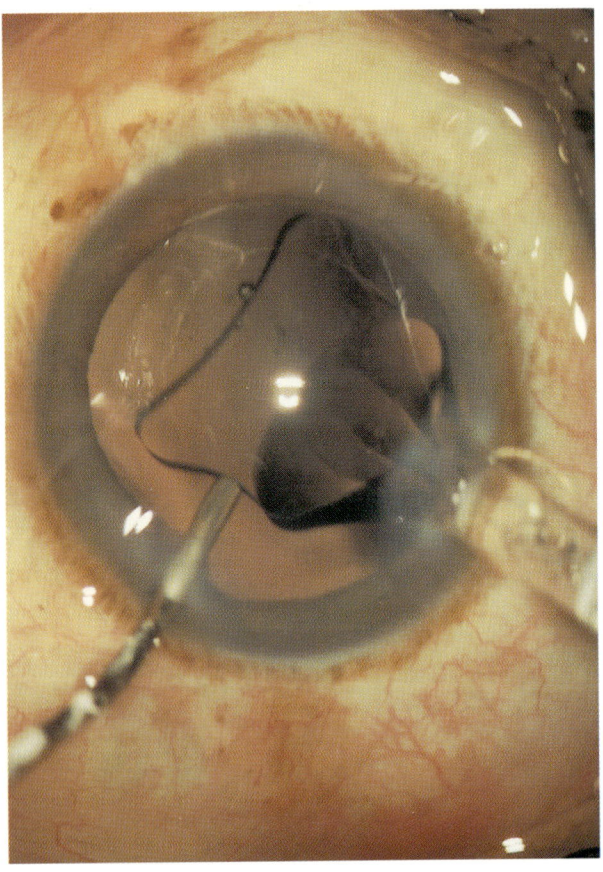

Figure 69: Acritec IOL implantation technique. The lens is loaded on to an injector and injected inside the eye.

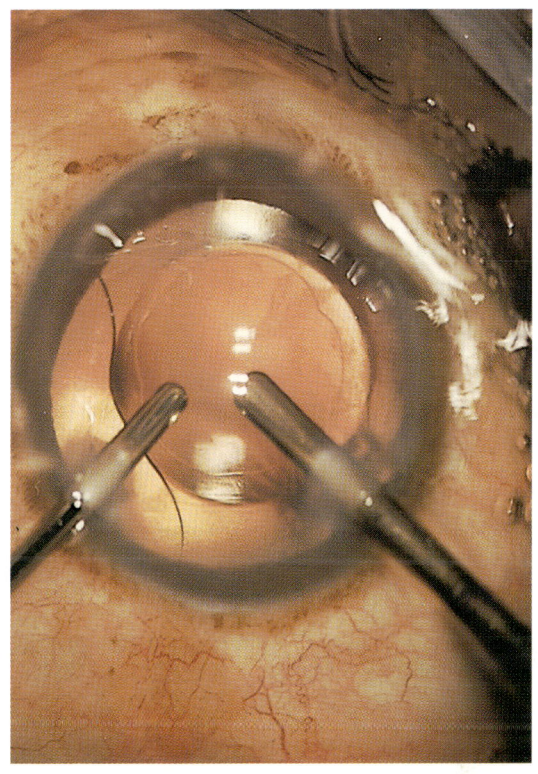

Figure 70: Acritec IOL implantation technique. The lens has unfolded inside the eye and is lying on the capsule.

What are the chances of good sight after Operation?

With the advancement of cataract surgery and modern skills, the success of cataract surgery is between 97 and 99%. Complications like infection and haemorrhage can occur but are very rare. One should remember that if the retina or the nerves of the eye are damaged even after a good cataract operation the person will not see.

Laser Surgery

Lasers have come a long way and nowadays everyone is talking about them. Lasers can be used to treat a primary cataract with the technique of **Laser Phakonit** or **Laser Phako**. Another cataract develops after sometime called an **After Cataract**. This cataract can be treated with the laser. When one operates a cataract, a capsule is left behind to help support the Intraocular lens. Sometimes, with time, after the cataract operation, this capsule thickens. (Fig. 71). This is called an After

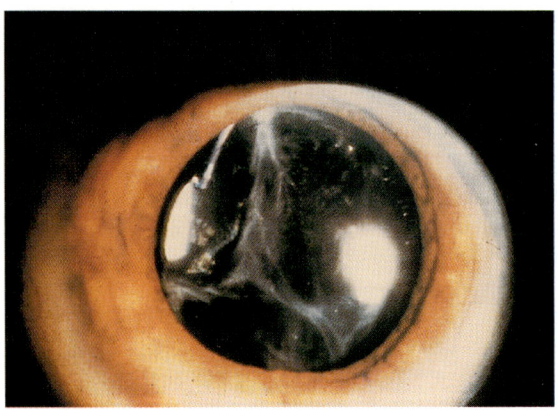

Figure 71: After cataract or secondary cataract. The capsule of the lens gets opacified and this is called an after cataract.

cataract. We can cut this with a small needle through a minor operation to make the vision clear again. This is again an operation and requires an injection and has the other problems of surgery. With the help of the laser called the **Yag Laser** (Fig. 72) this cataract can be removed as an outpatient treatment in 5 minutes. The procedure is absolutely painless.

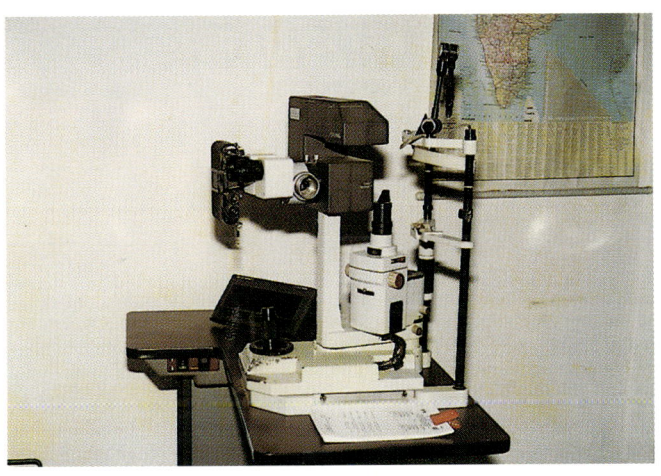

Figure 72: Yag Laser.

Glaucoma

What is Glaucoma?

Glaucoma is an eye disease which is one of the leading causes of blindness in our country. It is fairly common in adults above the age of 35 years. A clear transparent fluid called Aqueous humor flows through the inner eye continuously (Figs. 2 and 3). This inner flow can be compared to a sink with the tap turned on all the time. If the drainpipe gets blocked, water collects in the sink. Similarily in the eye there

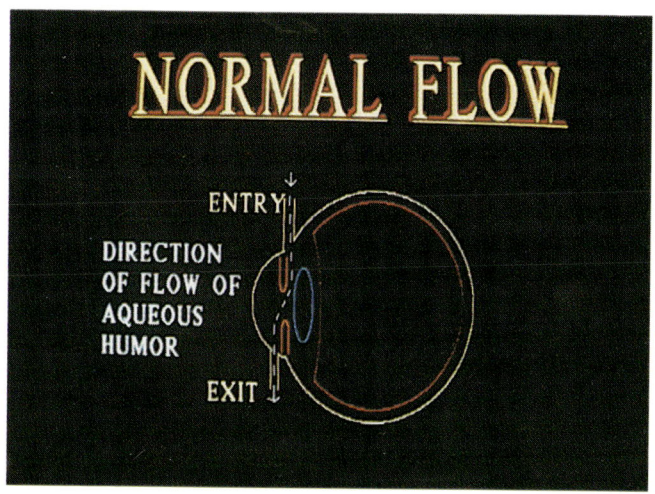

Figure 73: Normal draining of Aqueous Humor in the eye. The fluid flows in and out of the eye.

is a drainage system. Fluid is continuously coming into the eye and going out of the eye (Fig. 73). In Glaucoma, the fluid is entering the eye, but not going out because the drainage pipe of the eye is blocked (Fig. 74). Once this happens, the fluid accumulates in the eye and the pressure on the eye increases (Fig. 75). This increase in pressure indicates **Glaucoma**.

Why does Glaucoma affect Vision?

When we look at an object, the image is carried from the retina to the brain by the nerve of sight called the

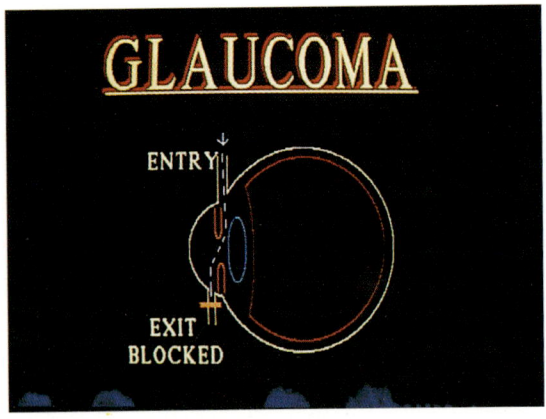

Figure 74: Glaucoma. If the exit is blocked then the pressure inside the eye increases, leading to glaucoma.

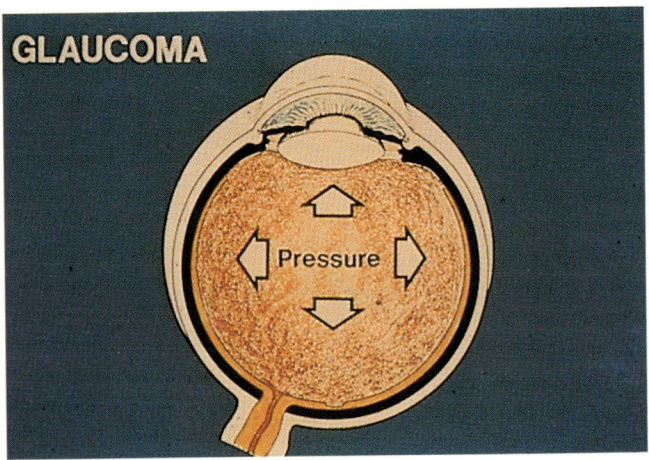

Figure 75: In glaucoma the pressure in the eye has increased. This causes pressure on the optic nerve of the eye. The optic nerve connects the retina to the brain.

Optic nerve (Figs. 2 and 3). Once the pressure builds up in the eye as in glaucoma this pressure compresses the optic nerve and starts to destroy it (Fig. 76). This produces a loss of vision. Imagine that we are watching a scenery, then due to the pressure on the optic nerve after sometime the sides will not be seen and slowly a patient with glaucoma sees only the central field of view. With the passage of time even this is lost. People seldom notice this until considerable damage has occurred. That is why glaucoma is called a thief in the night.

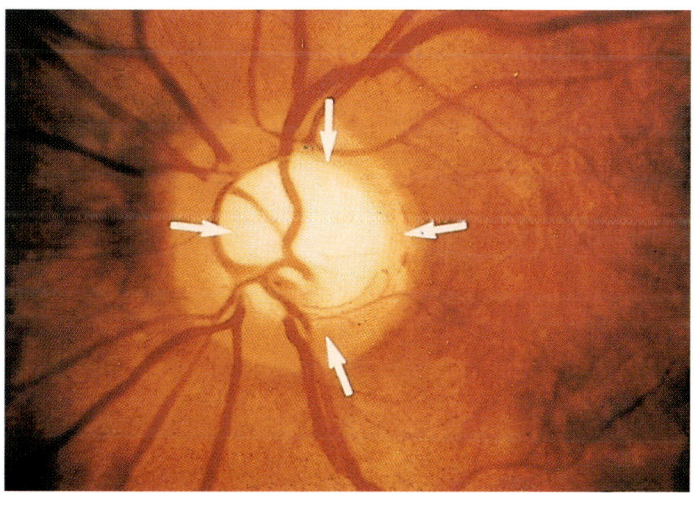

Figure 76: Once the pressure in the optic nerve has increased the nerve gets damaged and becomes more white as seen by the arrows in the figure. This is called cupping of the optic disc.

What are the Symptoms of Glaucoma?

1. Frequent changes of glasses, especially for near work, but none is satisfactory,
2. Rainbow coloured rings around lights,
3. Blurred or foggy vision and
4. Loss of side vision.

Keep in mind that having any of these symptoms does not necessarily mean that a person has glaucoma. It is better to get a check up of your eyes if you suffer from any of these symptoms.

Prevention of Glaucoma

Adults should see an eye doctor for periodic eye examinations. If there is a family history of glaucoma then one should be regular in the follow up. Early diagnosis can be made by the doctor testing your eye pressure on a specialised instrument, either with an **Applanation Tonometer or Non-contact Tonometer** (Fig. 21). These instruments are used to record the intraocular pressure. The field of vision can be tested on a machine called a **Autoperimeter** (Fig. 77). Remember that loss of vision already destroyed by glaucoma cannot be restored. So take care of your eyes, for they are very precious.

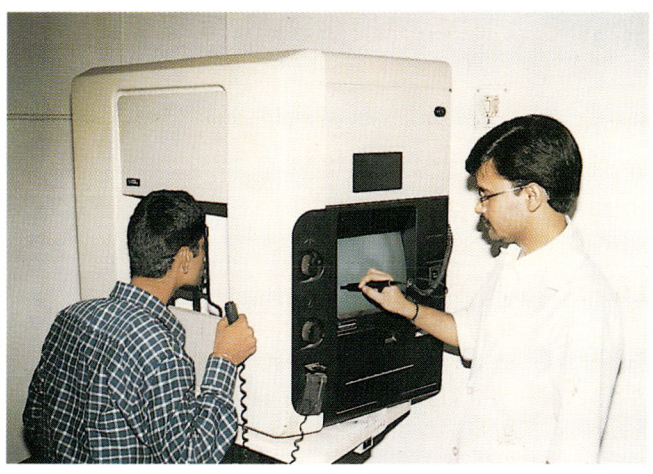

Figure 77: Autoperimeter. This is a computerised machine which tests the fields of the eye. In a glaucomatous patient the fields are constricted. In other words, the patient will not see the sides but will only see in the central areas.

Treatment

There are two ways to treat glaucoma. One, is to reduce the amount of fluid enetering the eye. This is done by drugs. The second is to open the block in the drainage pipe so that the fluid can go out easily. This is done by Lasers or by surgery.

Eye Transplantation

What is Eye Transplantation

The word eye transplantation is a misnomer because the whole eye can never be grafted. The cornea (Fig.2 and 3) is the front transparent window of the eye. It is through the cornea that light enters the eye and one is able to see. In some people, this window of the eye (cornea) gets diseased. In such cases, the only treatment is to remove their corneas and replace it or transplant it with a new healthy cornea of a dead person. This operation is called **Eye Transplantation** or **Corneal Transplantation** or **Corneal Grafting**.

Which Diseases Require Transplantation?

The normal cornea is spherical. In some people the cornea becomes conical. This is called **Conical Cornea** or **Keratoconus**. Such patients in the early stages benefit from contact lenses but later a corneal transplantation may be the only solution. Quite a number of eyes are lost due to injuries from bow and arrows or crackers. These eyes can get back vision with a corneal transplantation. Infections and chemical burns can also damage the cornea and vision can be restored with corneal transplantation.

Can a Living Person Donate Eyes?

No. Eyes are never taken from a living person. Once someone is dead, the relatives should contact an eye bank which will send a doctor to remove the eyes. Artificial eyes are fitted onto the deceased person so that the looks of the person are absolutely normal. Eyes from a dead person have to be removed within 6 hours of the death, otherwise the eyes are useless. The transplantation should be done as soon as possible. Sex is no bar for donating the eyes and even those who have had an eye operation done in their lives can donate. Death due to heart attacks, diabetes and tuberculosis do not prevent donation. There is also no age limit for eye donation.

Operation

Eyes collected from the dead person are stored in a moist chamber at 4 degrees centigrade and must be used for transplantation within 24 to 48 hours in patients suffering from corneal diseases. The surgery of corneal grafting is a sophisticated operation requiring a great deal of technical skill. The results are very good and the chances of success very high.

Squint

What is Squint?

Squint (Strabismus) is a condition in which there is a misalignment of the eyes. In other words, the two eyes are pointed in different directions. One eye may be pointing straight ahead while the other is turned inward, outward, upward or downward (Fig. 78). It is a common condition which affects 4% of children. It can occur later in life also, though the chances are less.

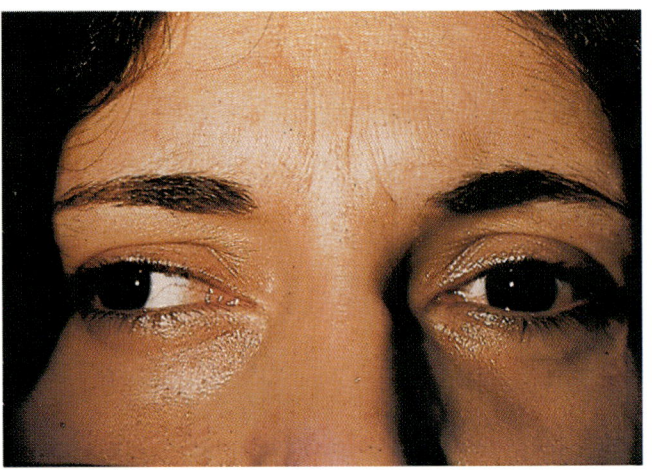

Figure 78: Squint. Note the right eye is deviated outwards and the left eye looks straight ahead.

Why does it Occur?

Our eye movements are controlled by our eye muscles (Fig 79). Imagine that one muscle is stronger than the other. The eye then will be turned towards that direction. This is how a squint is formed. To treat this, one has obviously to weaken the strong muscle and strengthen the weak muscle.

When should one get treated for Squint?

The treatment should be immediate. If one notices a squint, then an eye doctor should be consulted as soon

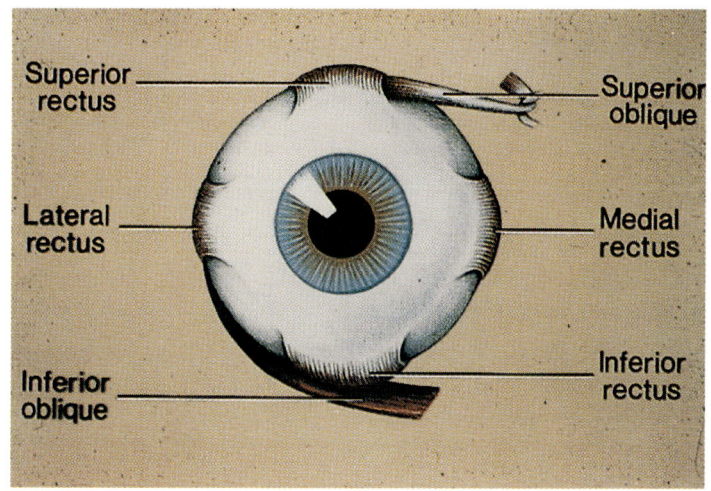

Figure 79: Muscles of the eye. The eye is moved by certain muscles and depending on them becoming weak or strong, squint occurs.

as possible. Parents often get the false impression that a child may "outgrow" the problem. Children never outgrow squint. Further, if the treatment is delayed after the age of 5 years, then the child will see only with one eye even after the squint is corrected. This is because till the age of 5 years both the eyes are developing and trying to work together. If a squint is there this cannot occur and only one eye works. After the age of 5 years even if the squint is corrected, only a cosmetic result can be achieved, but both the eyes can never work together.

Prevention

All eye defects of children should be treated as early as possible. While feeding babies with a bottle of milk, cover the bottle with a cloth so that the child does not make an effort to see the level of the milk in the bottle. Care should be taken to avoid exposure of the eyes of small infants to direct bright lights.

Treatment

The treatment can be either eye drops, spectacles, exercises or an operation. In the operation, the weak muscle is strengthened and the strong muscle is weakened.

Diabetes

What is Diabetes?

Diabetes mellitus is a condition which impairs the body's ability to use and store sugar. You get increased blood sugar, excessive thirst and increase in urine excretion.

What is Diabetic Retinopathy?

Diabetes may cause serious changes in the eye, like cataract and decreased vision. Diabetic retinopathy is a complication of diabetes that affects the eyes. In diabetic retinopathy damage occurs to the film of the eye called the retina (Figs. 2 and 3).

How does Diabetes damage the Retina?

The retina has a large number of blood vessels (Fig. 80) which give it nourishment. In diabetic retinopathy (Fig. 81), these vessels become weak. Once the vessels become weak, they start leaking fluid or

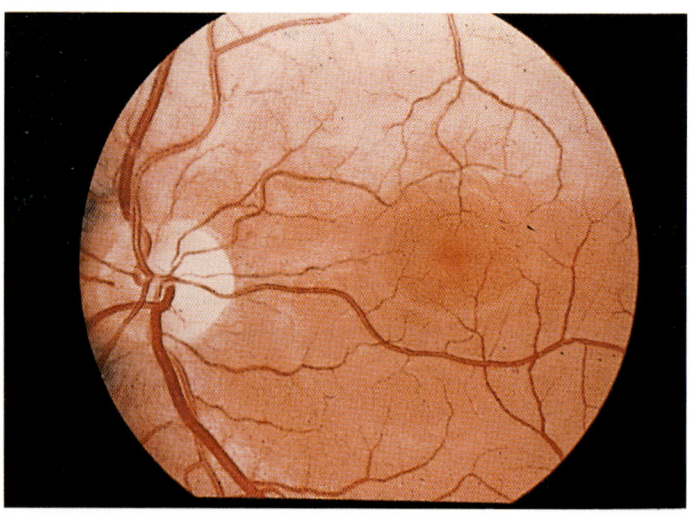

Figure 80: Normal retina. The retina is the film of the eye. Note that the white circular structure in the left is the optic disc which is the optic nerve of the eye. This connects the retina to the brain. Note that the red lines are the blood vessels of the retina.

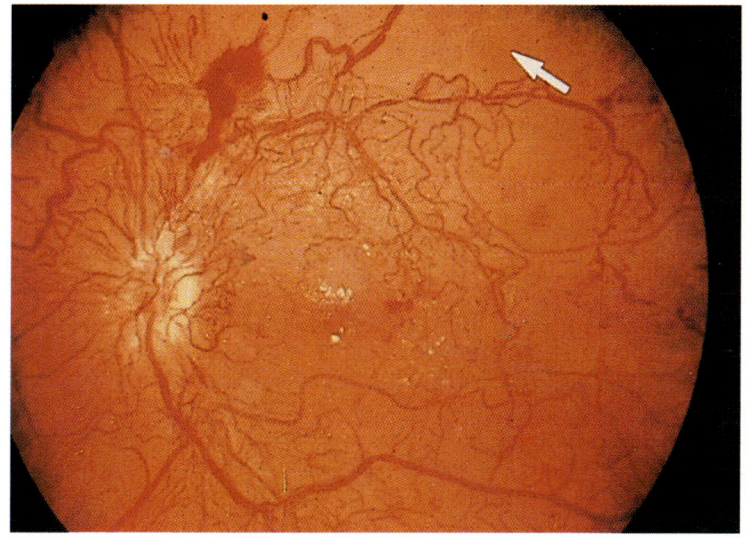

Figure 81: Diabetic Retinopathy. Notice the blood vessels have become tortuous and curved. These are new vessels which are defective and which will bleed.

blood. This leaking fluid or blood can damage the retina and when that happens the image sent to the brain gets blurred and the patient begins to lose vision.

Detection and Diagnosis

Diabetic patients must come regularly for a check up. An indirect ophthalmoscopic examination will detect diabetic retinopathy. To see which blood vessel is leaking, a **Fluorescein Angiograhy** test may be done (Fig. 82).

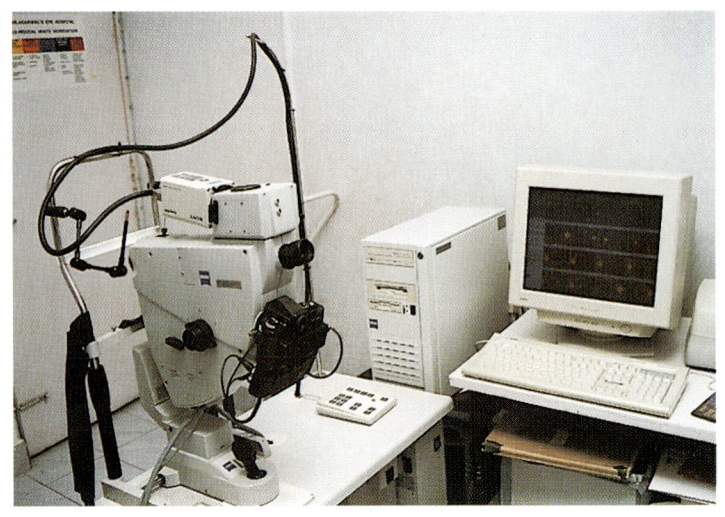

Figure 82: Digital Fluorescein Angiography Equipment.

In this, a fluorescent dye is injected into the patient's arm. This dye travels through the blood-stream and passes into the blood vessels of the retina. Photographs are taken rapidly as the dye leaks through the retina's blood vessels. This equipment has a special digital imaging system so the doctor can look at it any time later also. A printout of the photos is given to the patient.

Treatment

In early stages only control of the diabetes is enough. If the case is more advanced, **Laser Photocoagulation**

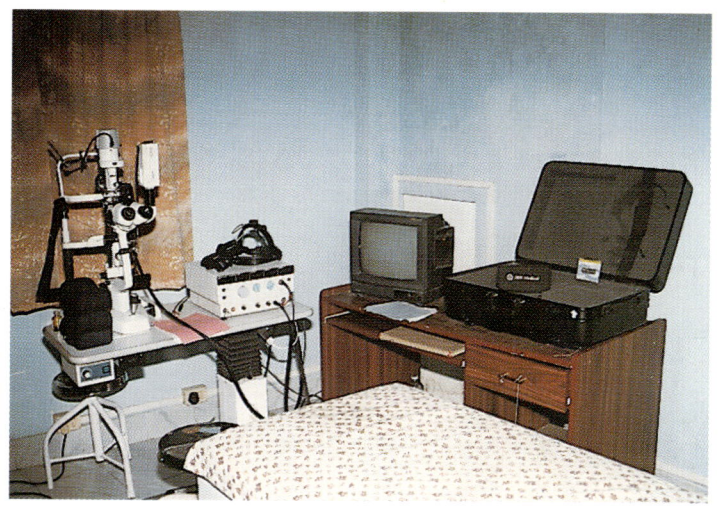

Figure 83: Argon laser machine.

may have to be done (Fig. 83). This procedure focuses a powerful beam of laser light onto the damaged retina to close the leaking vessels just as we do soldering. This procedure does not require any admission and is done on an out-patient basis. In the very late stages, if the retina has got seperated from its base and blood has collected in the eye, an operation in which a **Vitrectomy** (Fig. 84) and **Retinal Detachment Repair** has to be done.

In Vitrectomy the blood from inside the eye has to be removed. Three openings are made inside the eye.

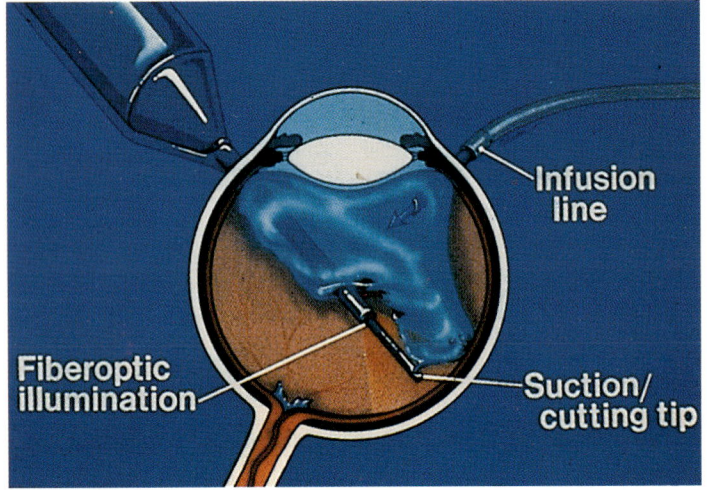

Figure 84: Vitrectomy. In this surgical technique the blood from inside the eye is removed. One line is the infusion line through which fluid passes into the eye to replace the blood which has filled inside the eye. The second instrument is the fiberoptic illumination which produces light inside the eye so that the surgeon can see what he is doing. The third instrument is the cutting and suction tip which cuts and sucks the blood inside the eye.

One opening is the infusion line through which fluid passes into the eye to replace the blood which has filled inside the eye. The second opening is for the fibe-roptic illumination which focuses light inside the eye so that the surgeon can see what he is doing. The third opening is for the instrument which does the cutting and suction. This cuts and sucks the blood inside the eye.

Retinal Detachment and other Retinal Diseases

What is Retinal Detachment?

In a normal eye, the retina which is the film of the eye is very close to the choroid which gives it nourishment (Figs. 2 and 3). In some people this retina gets separated from the choroid or in other words, it gets detached. This is called **Retinal Detachment**.

Why Does it Occur?

There are many causes of retinal detachment. The most common cause is short sight or myopia. When a person is short sighted or myopic, the person's eyeball is larger than normal. So, obviously, in a larger eyeball, the retina has to cover a larger surface area than normal. This it does by stretching. Due to this stretching the retina can tear at a particular place and lead to the formation of a retinal hole. Now vitreous fluid can enter through this hole and separate the retina from it's base (Fig. 85), leading to a retinal detachment.

Prevention of Retinal Detachment

As we have now understood the mechanism of formation of a retinal detachment, it is obvious that the precursor is a retinal hole. So, all myopic patients should have a thorough retinal examination every year to check if they have a retinal hole. If a retinal hole is detected, **Argon laser** (Fig. 83) treatment should be done to close the hole. This is absolutely painless, there is no injection and it is done as an out-patient treatment. It takes about 15 minutes. It is difficult for you to know if you have a retinal hole by yourself as there is no loss of vision. If you start to see black spots in front of your

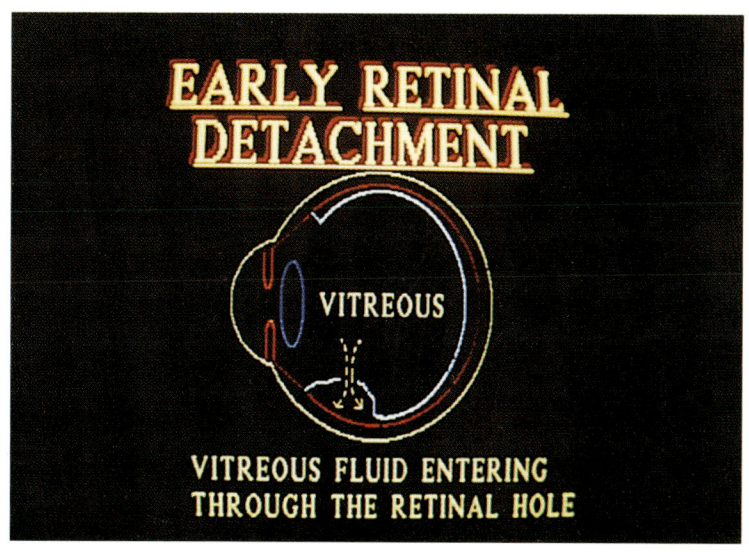

Figure 85: Early Retinal Detachment.

eyes or flashes of light then it could be due to the formation of a retinal hole and you should consult an eye doctor immediately.

Treatment of Retinal Detachment

The treatment of retinal detachment is surgery which is a major operation. That is why, one should try to prevent it's formation by getting a retinal hole treated.

Retinitis Pigmentosa

This is a developmental disease in which the patient has black pigments in the retina (Fig. 86). The patient does not see in the night. The patient should keep two tubelights in every room. This occurs specially when the parents have a consanguineous marriage, in other words are related by blood.

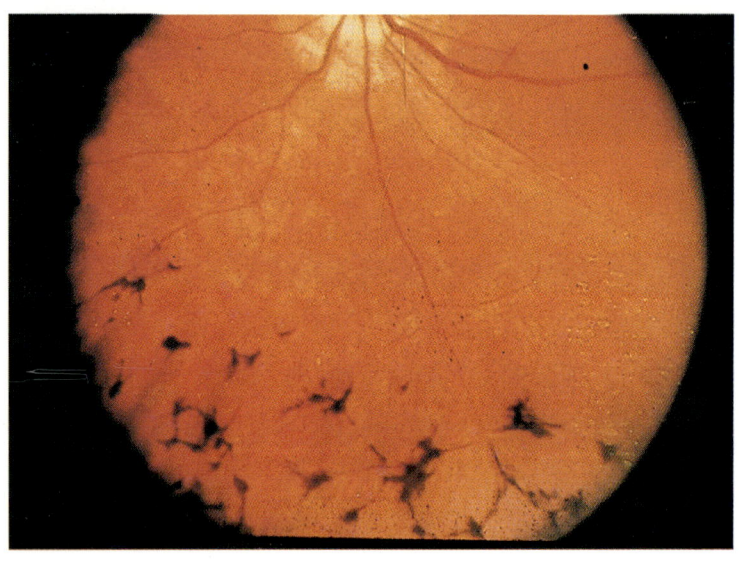

Figure 86: Retinitis Pigmentosa.
Notice the black pigments seen in the retina

Macular Degeneration

In Macular Degeneration (Fig. 87), the macula of the retina gets damaged with white spots which eventually leads to bleeding and scar formation. This occurs mainly due to an ageing process. The solution is to do Laser treatment or a Vitrectomy but the prognosis is very

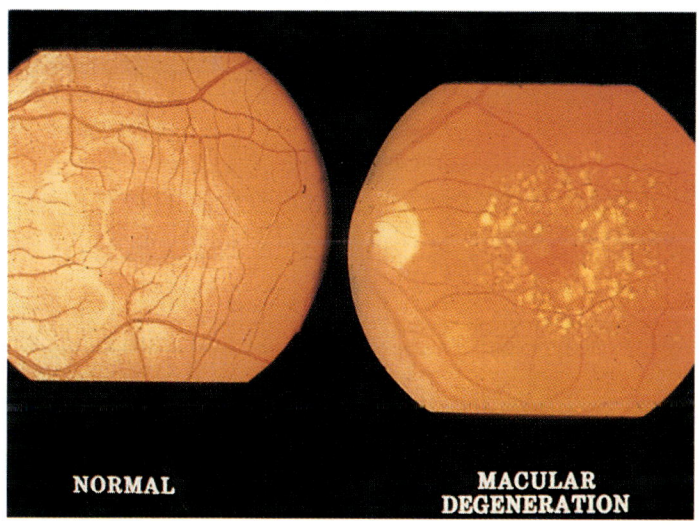

Figure 87: Macular Degeneration.

poor. To diagnose this condition in the early stages one should look at an **Amsler's grid** (Fig. 88). This is a chart with a central black spot and squares all around.

RE / LE

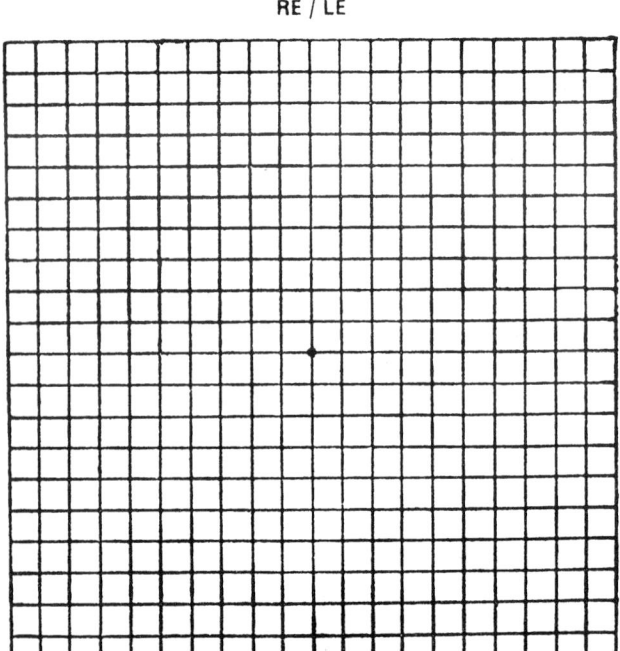

Figure 88: Amsler's grid. This is a chart with a central black spot and squares all around. Look at the central black spot with one eye keeping the other eye closed. Then note the lines. If they appear distorted or wavy consult an eye surgeon.

Look at the central black spot with one eye keeping the other eye closed. Then note the lines. If they appear distorted or wavy, consult an eye surgeon.

Injuries and Deficiency Diseases

Introduction

Injuries are common among children, especially caused by bows and arrows. Foreign bodies can also enter the eye. Crackers can also produce injury to the eye.

Prevention

The best method of preventing injuries in children is not to give them bows and arrows to play with. Do not give them guns with darts. Motorcycle riders should wear helmets with visors to prevent foreign bodies getting into their eyes. Children should not be allowed to play with crackers during Diwali.

Treatment

If a foreign body enters the eye, fill a cup with water. Now bring your eye towards the cup (Fig. 89). Let your eye be as close to the cup as possible and when the water touches your eye blink many times. If the foreign body is loose, it will get dislodged and come off. Even after this, if it does not come off, rush immediately to the nearest eye doctor. Major injuries might have to be operated upon.

Deficiency Diseases

In developing countries, the problem is poverty. This leads to undernourishment and deficency diseases. A child can suffer from various eye diseases as a result of lack of food. The earliest sign is white spots seen

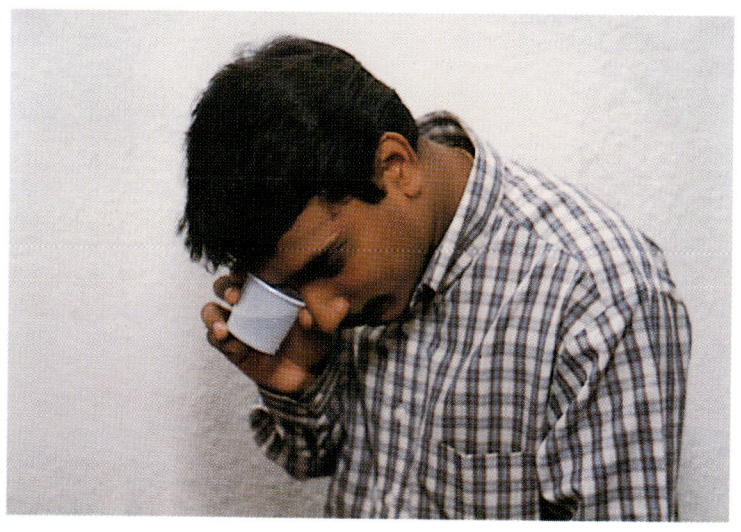

Figure 89: Treatment of a foreign body in the eye. Take a cup of water filled to the brim and bring it close to your eye. Blink repeatedly in the cup and most likely the foreign body will come out. If it does not then consult an eye doctor.

in the conjunctiva. These are called **Bitot's Spots**. The cornea can also start melting from deficiency of food. The prevention of this is to give the child good food with lots of vegetables and milk. Vitamins are necessary for the growth of the child. If one notices this in a child, the child should be taken to an eye doctor, who may give the child Vitamin A.

Hints

Hints for Mothers

1. Expectant mothers should make an effort to avoid contacting measles during the first two months of pregnancy.
2. Expectant mothers should avoid all medications as far as possible and use food supplements like vitamins and proteins.
3. If there is a discharge from the genital passages during pregnancy, inform the doctor and take

appropriate treatment to avoid the infection of the baby's eyes at birth.
4. Immediately after birth, wipe the baby's eyelids carefully with damp cotton-wool from the nose outwards before the eyes are opened.
5. A little bit of Erythromycin ointment applied as a routine to the baby's eyes at birth by the doctor or trained midwife practically eliminates a very important cause of blindness in children.
6. Water from the first bath should not be allowed to go into the baby's eyes.
7. If there is any discharge from the baby's eyes within the first seven days, consult an eye doctor immediately, otherwise it may result in loss of sight.
8. Do not expose the baby's eyes to direct strong light.
9. If the baby's eyes seem to be especially large towards the end of one month, consult an eye doctor as this is a sign of infantile glaucoma.

Hints for Teachers

1. Teach the proper use of eyes while reading, writing, etc.
2. A periodic eye test of school children is very important. An eye check up when the child joins the nursery class should be done.

3. If the child is not making proper progress in studies, the child may be visually defective.
4. Do not allow the children with sore eyes to mix and play with other children.
5. Make the children read a Snellen Test Chart every six months in the class room. The Snellen test chart is a chart to test the vision of a person (Fig.90).
6. At the time of leaving school, another eye test should be conducted for determining any defect of vision which might prevent the student's progress. Testing of colour vision is also important as colour blindness is a great handicap in certain occupations.

Hints for Adults

1. Protect yourself from sand, dust, smoke, etc.
2. Keep flies away as they are a source of infection.
3. Keep the house clean and develop healthy sanitary habits.
4. Never use common handkerchiefs, towels etc for wiping the eyes and face by the members of the same family.
5. Correct the habits of reading, writing, watching TV, etc.
6. Take care that the illumination for work is proper and adequate.

7. Industrial workers should use protective devices if their vocation demands so.
8. If there is an inflammation of the eye, immediate medical attention must be obtained.
9. In elderly persons, failing vision must be reported to the doctor.
10. If a foreign body gets in the eyes, it must be removed preferably by a doctor.
11. Marriages between cousins and near relations should always be avoided. It is estimated that the danger of blindness resulting from hereditary factors is 20 times higher among children of related parents than among those of ordinary marriages.
12. Never watch the solar-eclipse without protective glasses.

General Instructions

1. Rest your eyes periodically when doing prolonged close work.
2. Check all labels, expiry dates and directions on all medicines before instilling them in your eyes.
3. Wear appropriate protective eyewear while using, chemicals, welding arcs etc.
4. Flush your eyes with cold water in the event of a chemical injury.
5. Occasionally check your vision by covering one eye and then the other while looking at the Snellen's Visual Acuity Chart (Fig. 90).

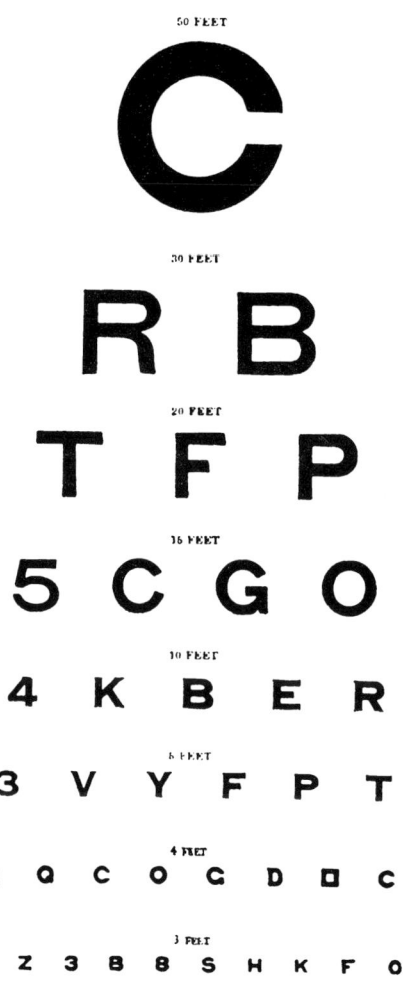

Figure 90: Snellen Visual Acuity Chart.

Important Signs and Symptoms

The following are important signs and symptoms that should prompt you to visit an eye doctor.

1. Sudden loss of vision or sudden blurred vision
2. Double vision.
3. Flashes of light or floaters in front of the eyes.
4. Sudden marked distortion of vision.

5. Severe redness of the eyes.
6. Severe pain in the eyes.
7. Any injury to the eyes.

Our Other Titles in Health:

BODY TALK
Dr Yatish Agarwal
Bodytalk discusses common ailments, their symptoms and management in a simple, direct and jargon-free style. From grandma's concoctions and remedies to the latest scientific discoveries, it sifts misconceptions and superstitions from hard truths and tells you how to safeguard against illnesses.

Dr Yatish Agarwal is a noted physician, writer and health columnist. His popular books, essays, articles, columns, radio broadcasts and T.V. serials have spread his message of good health and simple, sensible living to millions of people. He is a recipient of the Meghnad Saha Award (1991, '92 and '93) National Science Award (1988) and Atmaram Award (1993).

HINTS ON HEALTH
G.D. Thapar
Hints on Health attempts to help the reader gain better control over his health. Based on the latest advances in medicine and preventive health, it is designed to help him prevent some of the most serious diseases, which arise from a faulty lifestyle. Common diseases such as heart attacks, strokes, cirrhosis of the liver, common disorders such as hypertension and sexual dysfunction are described in detail and advice given

on how to deal with them.

A former Physician and Chief of Medical Unit at Willingdon (now RML) Hospital, New Delhi, and Consultant in Medicine and Cardiology at INAS Hospital, University of Tripoli, Dr G.D. Thapar, MD is the author of highly acclaimed books on medical subjects of his specialisation.

CURE AT HOME
N Anantharaman and A. Karthik

Ayurveda is the most ancient form of medicine and has its origin in India. The book underlines the advantages of the Ayurvedic way of life. It throws light on many home remedies that are time tested, simple and cost-effective, made out of ingredients easily available in the local *pansari* shop or our kitchen garden and are of invaluable use in tackling almost all the common ailments that can be thought of, from joint pain to cough and cold to indigestion to pimples!

Dr Anantha Raman is a post-graduate (M.D.) in Ayurveda from Bangalore University and has been practising Classical Ayurveda for almost two decades. He has more than 300 articles and successful books like *Mane Oushadhi*, *Arogya Margadarshi* and *Tonnu Chikitse* to his credit.

Dr A. Karthik is a meritorious medical graduate from the reputed Bangalore Medical College. He has published a number of articles on medical subjects in

Kannada and English newspapers. His book *Liver Disorders* has been widely appreciated.

PLANTS FOR GOOD HEALTH
Manisha Jain
This book elucidates the medicinal and curative properties of common plants. It enlists the nutritive elements present in various plants and also gives simple recipes for making various decoctions and home-cures. For instance, apples and grapes not only taste good but also give you a good eyesight and increase your resistance to diseases.
Manisha Jain is a journalist who specialises in health, education and gender issues.

A GUIDE TO HOMOEOPATHIC REMEDIES: THE COMPLETE MODERN HANDBOOK FOR HOME USE
Paul Houghton
Homeopathic remedies are among the safest medicines you can take–gentle, effective and completely natural. This practical and amazingly comprehensive book, written by a practicing homoeopath, explains all about the what, when and who of homoeopathy.

YOGA FOR BUSY PEOPLE
Bijoylaxmi Hota
Yoga For Busy People is a user friendly book containing information necessary for maintaining good health, especially of a busy person who is likely to lose it the

most.

Apart from recommending the most simple yogic techniques that can be practised with ease by anyone, the book also shows how to fit them all into one's busy schedule.

Bijoylaxmi Hota is a Yoga Therapist of repute with almost two and a half decades of experience.

NATURALLY BEAUTIFUL: YOUR FACE

Naturally Beautiful is a tribute: a tribute to the beauty, culture and tradition of Indian womanhood. A culture that has been known for the simplicity of its principles and one whose roots are buried in age old tradition. Indian beauty has now come into its own and is duly recognized the world over for its calm intrinsic wholeness.

Face - the most arresting feature of a person-needs just a little care and attention to radiate health and confidence. This book will show you how to bring the glow back to your face and erase the ravages of time and pollution.

NATURALLY BEAUTIFUL: YOUR HAIR

Women of rare beauty have always been associated with thick, long, lustrous and flowing hair. The hair is the final crowning glory. This book unravels the secret of thick, beautiful hair with some simple yet time tested hair-care routines.

NATURALLY BEAUTIFUL: YOUR SKIN

Soft and smooth skin and well-sculpted hands have always sent poets into raptures. The skin, hands and feet need special care and treatment to deal with ravages of the environment. This book unfolds age-old potions and remedies that keep them pampered and young.

Ambika Manchanda began her journalistic career three decades ago with *The Times of India*. She was the sub-editor with the *Sunday Times* and thereafter as a reporter with the *Economic Times*. She has published more than a thousand articles both in English and Hindi.

PREGNANCY

By Nutan Pandit

This book tells you all about childbirth, answering questions on weight gain, proper diet, exercises, breathing patterns, positions to adopt during labour, post-natal care of both mother and child and sex during and after pregnancy.

Nutan Pandit is a well-known pregnancy expert who started taking natural childbirth classes in 1978. She has visited the National Childbirth Trust in London and attended their classes and workshops. She now takes such classes at her home in New Delhi.